Workbook

Laboratory Testing *for* Ambulatory Settings: A Guide for Health Care Professionals

Second Edition

Marti Garrels, MSA, MT (ASCP), CMA (AAMA)
Medical Assisting Program Director
Lake Washington Technical College
Kirkland, Washington

Carol S. Oatis, MSEd, MT SM (ASCP), CMA (AAMA)
Microbiology Adjunct Instructor
Lake Sumter Community College
Leesburg, Florida

ELSEVIER
SAUNDERS

ELSEVIER
SAUNDERS

3251 Riverport Lane
St. Louis, Missouri 63043

WORKBOOK FOR LABORATORY TESTING FOR AMBULATORY SETTINGS: A GUIDE FOR HEALTH CARE PROFESSIONALS ISBN: 978-1-4377-1908-6

ISBN-13: 978-1-4377-1908-6

Executive Editor: Susan Cole
Developmental Editor: Jennifer Bertucci
Publishing Services Manager: Catherine Jackson
Senior Project Manager: David Stein
Project Manager: Priya Dauntess
Design Direction: Teresa McBryan

Printed in the United States of America

Last digit is the print number: 9 8 7 6 5 4 3

Contents

Introduction

This workbook is designed to build mastery over the highly technical and fascinating field of laboratory medicine. Most chapters are organized into five sections: terminology exercises; review questions for fundamental concepts, procedures, advanced concepts; and check-off procedure sheets for all the procedures presented in the textbook chapter. The completed workbook exercises and check-off procedure sheets fulfill all the competency objectives listed at the beginning of each chapter in the textbook. The appendix of the workbook contains laboratory maintenance logs, report forms, quality control logs, patient logs, and a sample health screening assessment form. These forms provide the documentation needed to prove laboratory quality assurance, safety compliance, and proper charting of test results.

TIPS FOR MASTERING EACH CHAPTER

Terminology Exercises

Before reading each chapter, you should become familiar with the technical terms related to the subject. The Evolve Web site provides tutorial exercises using these terms, and the matching exercises in this workbook can help you learn the terms. Making flashcards of the terms is also recommended. As you read the text and fill in your structured notes (from the Evolve Web site), you will find each of the terms bolded and defined in context to reinforce and build further understanding.

Basic Concepts, Procedures, and Advanced Concepts: Review Questions and Labeling

The questions, pictures, and diagrams in these three sections fulfill the stated objectives for each chapter. The questions are designed to follow the textbook and structured notes from the Evolve Web site. You are encouraged to use the textbook alongside the workbook for visual reinforcement and as a reference for finding data from the tables and flow charts. The advanced concepts sections contain complex critical-thinking exercises, as well as referencing detailed laboratory test information in chapters 3 through 9. Your course instructor may assign one or more of these three sections, depending on the time frame of the course.

Check-off Procedure Sheets

The outcome-based procedure sheets are found at the end of each chapter. You are encouraged to locate in the textbook the corresponding procedure box, which provides pictures of the steps involved in each procedure. The procedures fall into two categories: *Skill Procedures,* such as using a microscope, instructing patients, collecting specimens, and staining slides, and *Analytical Tests* in which you follow a test procedure to obtain test results, such as urinalysis, hemoglobin, glucose, and strep tests. In both cases, it is essential that you read, perform, and check off each step on the sheet as satisfactory or unsatisfactory. The steps marked with an asterisk (*) are critical for demonstrating competency. The *Skill Procedures* usually are performed with the instructor verifying each step. The *Analytical Tests* may be performed with a laboratory partner verifying the steps leading up to the test result. The instructor then verifies the final test result and the proper documentation of the test result to fulfill the required measurable outcome.

1 Introduction to the Laboratory and Safety Training

VOCABULARY REVIEW

Match each definition with the correct term.

_______ 1. Most of the population will test within a range of similar results when testing an analyte

_______ 2. Laboratory orders indicating what tests are to be done

_______ 3. A steady state of internal chemical and physical balance

_______ 4. The substance being tested, such as glucose or cholesterol, in a body specimen

_______ 5. A test result indicating a threat to a patient's health

_______ 6. The patient's willingness to follow the treatment plan and take an active role in his or her own health care

_______ 7. Tests that provide simple, unvarying results and require a minimal amount of judgment and interpretation

_______ 8. Clotting ability of blood

_______ 9. A facility or an area within a medical setting in which materials or specimens from the human body are examined or analyzed

_______ 10. The inability to regulate blood sugar levels

_______ 11. Long-lasting, debilitating conditions

_______ 12. Disease-causing microorganisms

_______ 13. Outpatient health care setting in which patients are not bedridden

A. diabetes mellitus
B. homeostasis
C. reference range
D. pathogens
E. compliance
F. CLIA waived tests
G. chronic disorders
H. analyte
I. critical value
J. ambulatory care
K. requisitions
L. coagulation
M. clinical laboratory

Identify the following acronyms.

14. POCT ____

15. CBC ____

16. POL ____

FUNDAMENTAL CONCEPTS

Overview of the Laboratory

17. List the three reasons a physician would prescribe a laboratory test.

____

____

____

18. List the three ways a specimen is analyzed.

____

____

____

19. List the three types of medical laboratories.

____

____

____

20. List three examples of professional credentials (or titles) obtained by individuals who perform laboratory tests based on their educational background (see Table 1-1 in the textbook).

Doctorate: 8 or more years of education	Master: 6 or more years of education	Bachelor: 4 or more years of education	Associate: 1 to 2 years of education

21. List three important characteristics required of laboratory personnel.

____

____

____

22. Give three reasons why a physician would want a test performed in the office and three reasons the specimen would be tested at an outside laboratory.

Advantages of In-Office Testing	Advantages of Out-of-Office Testing

23. From the reference laboratory requisition form (see Figure 1-6 in the textbook), write the first three laboratory tests listed in the following categories for blood, and provide the procedure code and blood collection container.

Test Category	Reference Laboratory Tests (see Requisition)	CPT Code (Left of Test)	Container (Right of Test)
Hematology tests			
Chemistry tests			
Serology/immunology tests			

24. Give the metric unit and abbreviation for each basic unit of measurement.

Measurement	Metric Unit	Abbreviation
Weight		
Length		
Volume (capacity)		

25. Give the metric prefix and abbreviation for each of the following.

Fractions	Prefix	Abbreviation
1/10, or 0.1		
1/100, or 0.01		
1/1000, or 0.001		
1/1,000,000, or 0.000001		

26. The following laboratory supplies have temperature storage directions on them. Where should they be stored?

Store at 15° to 30° C ______________________

Store at 0° C ______________________

Store at 4° to 8° C ______________________

27. Give the military times for the following Greenwich times.

3:00 PM ______________________

8:35 AM ______________________

9:15 PM ______________________

Noon ______________________

Safety Training

_______ 28. A documented plan provided by a facility to eliminate or minimize occupational exposure to bloodborne pathogens

_______ 29. Danger related to the exposure to toxic, unstable, explosive, or flammable materials

_______ 30. A means of transporting an infectious agent or pathogen from the infected individual to another by air, food, hand-to-hand contact, insects, or body fluids

_______ 31. The assumption that the blood or body fluid containing blood from any patient or test kit could be infectious

_______ 32. A disease that is spread within a health care facility

_______ 33. Federal law protecting employees' right to know about the dangers of the hazardous chemicals they may be exposed to under normal working conditions

_______ 34. Through the skin

_______ 35. An area that has been in contact with materials or environmental surfaces where infectious organisms may reside

_______ 36. Specialized clothing or equipment worn by an employee for protection against infectious materials

_______ 37. Efforts and research toward isolating and removing bloodborne pathogens from the workplace

_______ 38. Danger related to exposure to infectious and bloodborne pathogens

_______ 39. Dangers related to electricity, fire, weather emergencies, bomb threats, and accidental injuries

_______ 40. Policies that are recorded, monitored, and evaluated to protect employees from exposure to the pathogens in blood or body fluids

_______ 41. Putting on clothing or equipment as a barrier to a hazard

_______ 42. CDC recommendations for infection control in health facilities

A. chemical hazard
B. standard precautions
C. nosocomial infection (HCAI)
D. exposure control plan
E. percutaneous
F. work practice controls
G. universal precautions
H. donning personal protective equipment
I. transmission
J. physical hazards
K. engineering controls
L. personal protective equipment
M. hazard communication standard
N. contaminated
O. biohazards

43. List three ways that pathogens (infectious organisms) are transmitted.

____

____

____

44. List three methods to sanitize hands. (Hint: Each uses a different cleanser.)

____

____

____

45. Label the following personal protective equipment.

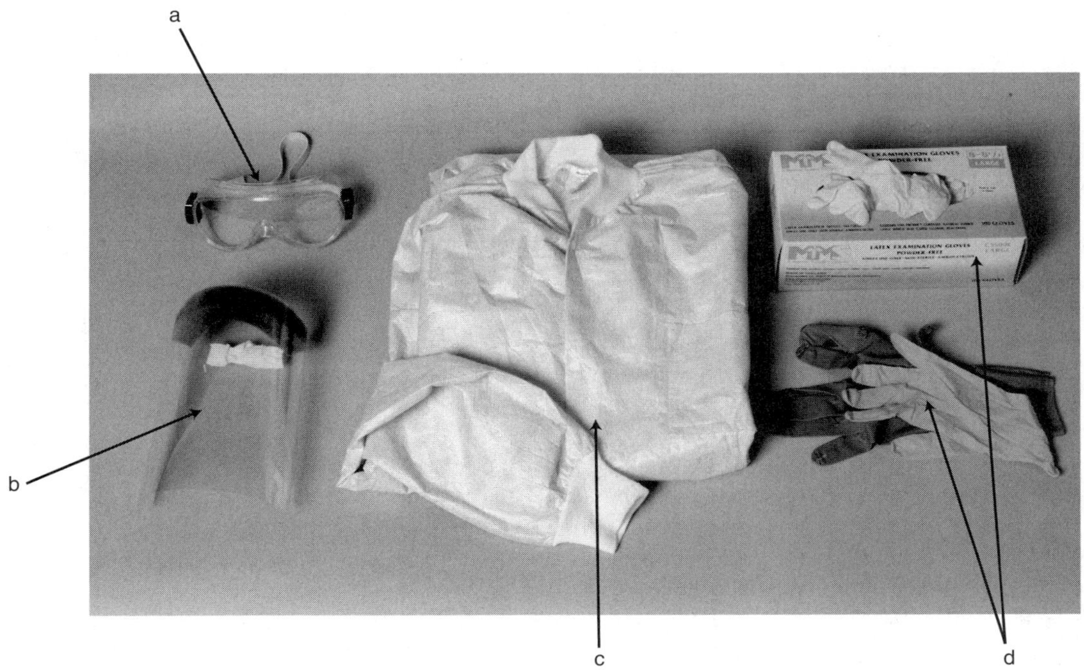

46. In which of the following disposal containers would contaminated gloves be disposed: wastebasket, biohazard waste container, or biohazard sharps container?

____

47. List the three major bloodborne pathogens. (Hint: They are all viral.)

____

____

____

48. Identify the following acronyms related to the bloodborne pathogen standard.

HCAIs ______________________________

OPIM ______________________________

PPE ______________________________

PEP ______________________________

49. Identify the following acronyms related to chemical hazard training.

MSDS ____________________

NFPA ____________________

HMIS ____________________

50. List three safety rules that must be observed in the laboratory, and explain why.

____

____

____

51. Use the Internet to locate and identify any OSHA or CDC updates on laboratory safety.

____

Laboratory Safety Checklist

Tour the laboratory with the safety checklist below and perform the bloodborne pathogen training posttest after the tour.

Item	Located
Physical safety	
First-aid kit	
Fire extinguisher	
Evacuation routes	
Fire	
Tornado	
Other (bomb threat)	
Chemical safety items	
Eyewash station	
Material Safety Data Sheets (MSDS)	
Caustic spill kit (if needed)	
Acid spill kit (if needed)	
Hazardous labeling	
Biologic safety items	
Bleach disinfectant	
Biohazard spill kit	
Sharps container	
Biohazard container	
Hand sanitizing stations	
Safety devices on needles and lancets	
Personal protective equipment	
Gloves	
Eye goggles and face shields	
Laboratory coat/gown, liquid impenetrable	
Documentation resources	
MSDS/safety manual	
Maintenance logs	
Quality control and patient logs	
Laboratory procedure manual	

OSHA Bloodborne Pathogen Quiz

1. A laboratory worker exposed to potentially infectious materials on the job may request a vaccine for which bloodborne disease?
   A. HIV
   B. syphilis
   C. hepatitis B
   D. brucellosis

2. Which of the following materials could contain bloodborne pathogens?
   A. bloody saliva
   B. semen
   C. vaginal secretions
   D. all the above

3. If gloves are worn when cleaning up an accident site, washing the hands afterward is not necessary.
   A. true
   B. false

4. Bloodborne pathogens may enter the system through
   A. open cuts
   B. skin abrasions
   C. dermatitis
   D. mucous membranes
   E. all the above

5. All body fluids should be treated as infectious, and direct skin contact with them should be avoided.
   A. true
   B. false

6. Eating, drinking, and smoking should never take place in a laboratory or other area where potential exposure to bloodborne pathogens exists.
   A. true
   B. false

7. What should be done *first* after an exposure incident?
   A. file an exposure report
   B. wash the exposed area
   C. find out if the patient is infected
   D. consult a physician

8. Waste that is dripping blood must be placed in containers that are color coded or clearly labeled "biohazard."
   A. true
   B. false

9. A 10% solution of one part household bleach to nine parts water provides a strong enough solution to decontaminate most surfaces, tools, and equipment effectively if left for 10 minutes.
   A. true
   B. false

10. How can puncture wounds be avoided?
    A. discard used disposable needles in the appropriate container
    B. do *not* recap used needles (use safety activated devices)
    C. practice using safety devices before using on patients
    D. all the above

Procedure 1-1: Proper Use of Personal Protective Equipment

Person evaluated ______________________________ Date ______________

Evaluated by ______________________________ Score ______________

Outcome goal	Demonstrate the proper use of personal protective equipment
Conditions	Given the following supplies: hand sanitizer nonpowdered gloves fluid-impenetrable gowns with cuffs at the wrists face masks and goggles, or full face shield (if the procedure to be performed has the potential for splashing)
Standards	Required time: 10 minutes Performance time ________ Total possible points = ________ Points earned = ________
Evaluation Rubric Codes: **S** = Satisfactory, meets standard **U** = Unsatisfactory, fails to meet standard	

Preparation	**Scores S**	**Scores U**
1. Before **donning** (putting on) PPE, remember to perform the hand wash or hand rub appropriately.		
Procedure	**S**	**U**
2. Follow the proper sequence for donning PPE.		
a. Put on the gown.		
b. Put on any face protectors.		
c. Don disposable nonsterile, nonpowdered, nonlatex, well-fitting gloves.		
d. Extend the gloves over the gown cuffs.		
3. Keep gloved hands away from the face. Remove gloves if they become torn, and perform hand hygiene before donning new gloves. Avoid touching other surfaces and items not involved in the testing process. The outside of the front of the gown is considered contaminated. The "clean" areas of the gown and gloves are on the inside and the back of the gown.		
4. Sequence for removing PPE:		
a. Properly take off gloves as follows:		
Remove one glove by grasping the outside with the other gloved hand and pulling it off.		
Wad up the removed glove in the gloved hand. Slip an ungloved finger under the cuff and fold it over until you can grasp the inside area of the second glove.		
Pull off the second glove inside-out with the first glove still inside.		
b. Remove the face shield.		
c. Remove the gown.		

Follow-up	Scores	
	S	U
5. If the gloves have visible blood or body fluid on them, dispose of them in a biohazard waste receptacle.		
6. Perform hand hygiene (hand wash or hand rub) immediately after removing PPE.		
Total Points per Column		

2 Regulations, Microscope Setup, and Quality Assurance

VOCABULARY REVIEW

Match each definition with the correct term.

_______ 1. Tests that produce a result measured as a number

_______ 2. A substance or ingredient used in a laboratory test to detect, measure, examine, or produce a reaction

_______ 3. An *overall* process to aid in improving the reliability, efficiency, and quality of laboratory test results

_______ 4. Materials with known values of the substance measured that help the laboratory achieve accurate and reliable testing by checking if the test system is working

_______ 5. Instructions included by the manufacturer located in the kit or test package

_______ 6. Proving competency by testing a specimen from an outside accreditation agency

_______ 7. Tests that simply look for the presence or absence of a substance

_______ 8. A process in which known samples (controls) are routinely tested to establish the reliability, accuracy, and precision of a specific test system

_______ 9. All components of a test that are packaged together

_______ 10. A built-in positive control to prove the device or test kit is working

_______ 11. The awareness and prevention of both the physical and procedural risks that may bring about an injury or legal action against the practice

_______ 12. A pattern of narrow and wide bars and spaces; each pattern is encoded with its own particular meaning

_______ 13. When both accuracy and precision are accomplished

_______ 14. Liquid positive and negative controls that are tested the same way as the liquid patient specimen

_______ 15. Ability to produce the same test result each time a test is performed (results are seen clustered together on a target)

_______ 16. The average test result of a series of controls

_______ 17. A statistical term describing the amount of variation from the mean in a dataset

_______ 18. When controls consistently fall within the two standard deviations of the mean (results are seen within the center of a target)

_______ 19. Used to plot the daily results of the control samples

A. package insert
B. quality assurance
C. qualitative
D. quality control
E. kit
F. quantitative
G. reagent
H. proficiency testing
I. controls
J. accuracy
K. Levy-Jennings chart
L. medical office risk management
M. bar codes
N. reliability
O. standard deviation
P. precision
Q. internal control
R. external controls
S. mean

GOVERNMENT ACRONYMS WORKSHEET

As you write the words for each government acronym or abbreviation, notice its relationship to the various divisions of government and its effect on ambulatory laboratories.

Federal departments	HHS =				Department of Labor	
Divisions within the department	OCR = Office of Civil Rights	CMS =	FDA =	CDC =	OSHA =	
Laws and/or regulations affecting laboratories	HIPAA: OCR enforces privacy standards	HIPAA: CMS enforces insurance portability		Infection control:	Infection control, blood:	Hazard communication standard
		CLIA: CMS administers the laboratory certifications	CLIA: FDA classifies laboratory test complexity	CDC recommends standard precautions for all infectious diseases	OSHA regulates BBPS =	OSHA regulates chemical hazards
Additional acronyms and abbreviations	HIPAA = PHI =	CLIA = QA = QC =	CoW = PPM =		PPE = OPIM = PEP =	MSDS = HMIS = NFPA =
Additional notes						

CLIA Government Regulations

20. What is the purpose of the Clinical Laboratory Improvement Amendment (CLIA 1988), and how does it benefit the patient?

____

____

21. What are the three categories of testing under CLIA, and under which category is physician-performed microscopy listed?

____

____

____

22. Review Table 2-1 in the textbook, which lists most of the CLIA-waived tests available. Locate three tests in each category, and list their corresponding procedure codes on the chart:

Test Category	Physician Office Tests	Procedure Code (CPT; 5-digit code)
Hematology tests		
Blood chemistry tests		
Serology/immunology tests		
Microbiology tests (only two)		

23. From the provider-performed microscopy procedure in Table 2-2 in the textbook, write the procedure codes for each of the following:

    a. Wet mounts, including preparations of vaginal, cervical, or skin specimens ______________

    b. Urinalysis (microscopic only) ______________

    c. All potassium hydroxide preparations ______________

24. Label the microscope, and perform the microscopic procedure at the end of the chapter.

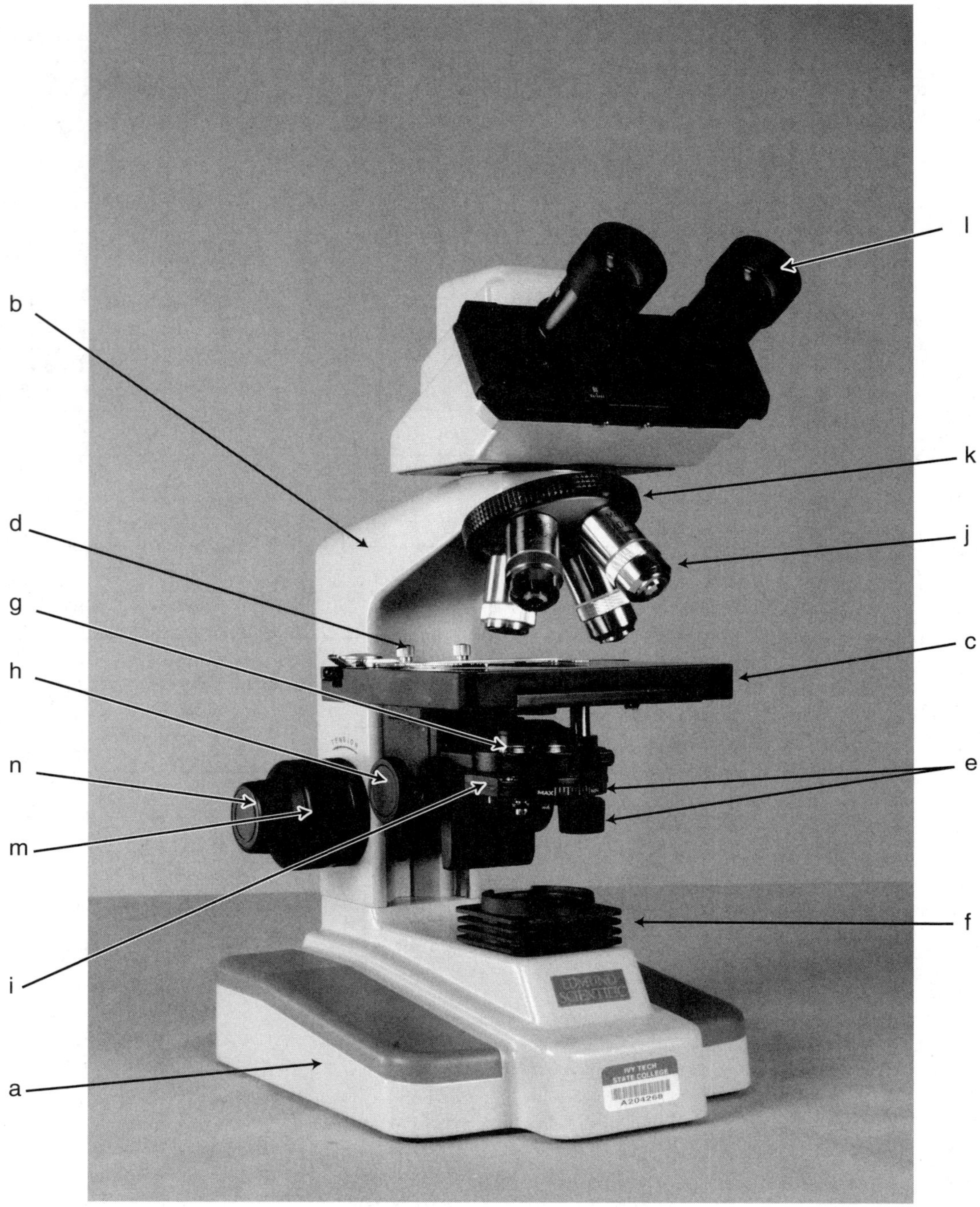

25. List three structures under each of the functional areas of the microscope.

Foundational	**Illuminating**	**Magnifying**
a. ______	a. ______	a. ______
b. ______	b. ______	b. ______
c. ______	c. ______	c. ______

GOOD LABORATORY PRACTICES

Quality Assurance

26. Compare the 10 areas of good laboratory practices for certificate of waiver laboratories (Figure 2-2 in the textbook) with the flow chart of the three phases of laboratory testing requiring quality assessment (Table 2-3 in the textbook). Draw lines between the good laboratory practices numbers to divide the three phases of preanalytical, analytical, and postanalytical. Where should the lines be placed?

______

______

27. Quality assurance oversees what areas of good laboratory practices? Quality control takes place during what areas of good laboratory practices?

______

______

28. What is the difference between qualitative tests and quantitative tests, and how does it affect quality control?

______

______

______

29. Explain the relationship of accuracy, precision, and reliability when plotting the results of standard controls.

______

______

______

______

HIPAA Privacy Rule, Risk Management, Electronic Medical Records, and Bar Coding

30. Are laboratory personnel allowed to give an interested party a patient's test results? Why or why not? Base the answer on the Health Insurance Portability and Accountability Act (HIPAA) and risk management principles of avoiding financial and legal consequences.

____

____

____

____

31. What is the single most important use of bar codes in the medical laboratory?

____

____

32. Plot 4 weeks of daily glucose control results on the four blank Levy-Jennings graphs. Mark the results for each day on the graph, and in the blank provided, identify whether the test system is experiencing a *trend,* a *shift,* a *random error,* or is *out of control.*

WEEK 1: day 1 = 103, day 2 = 100, day 3 = 98, day 4 = 112, day 5 = 105, day 6 = 99

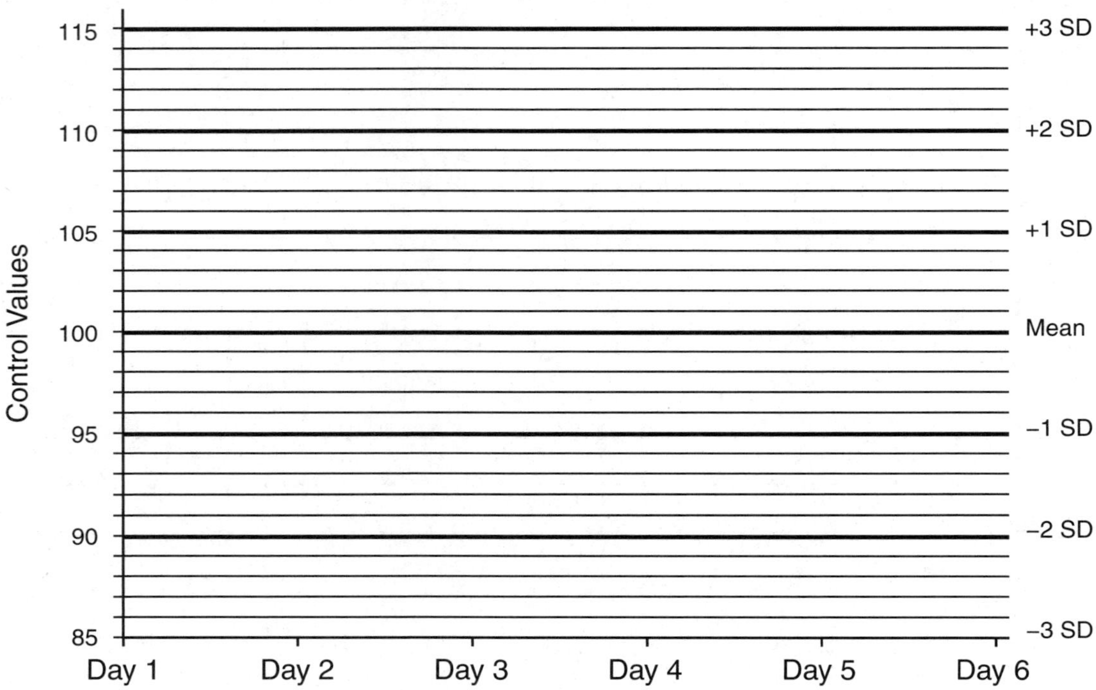

Week 1 glucose control results: ____________________

WEEK 2: day 1 = 94, day 2 = 92, day 3 = 93, day 4 = 108, day 5 = 109, day 6 = 107

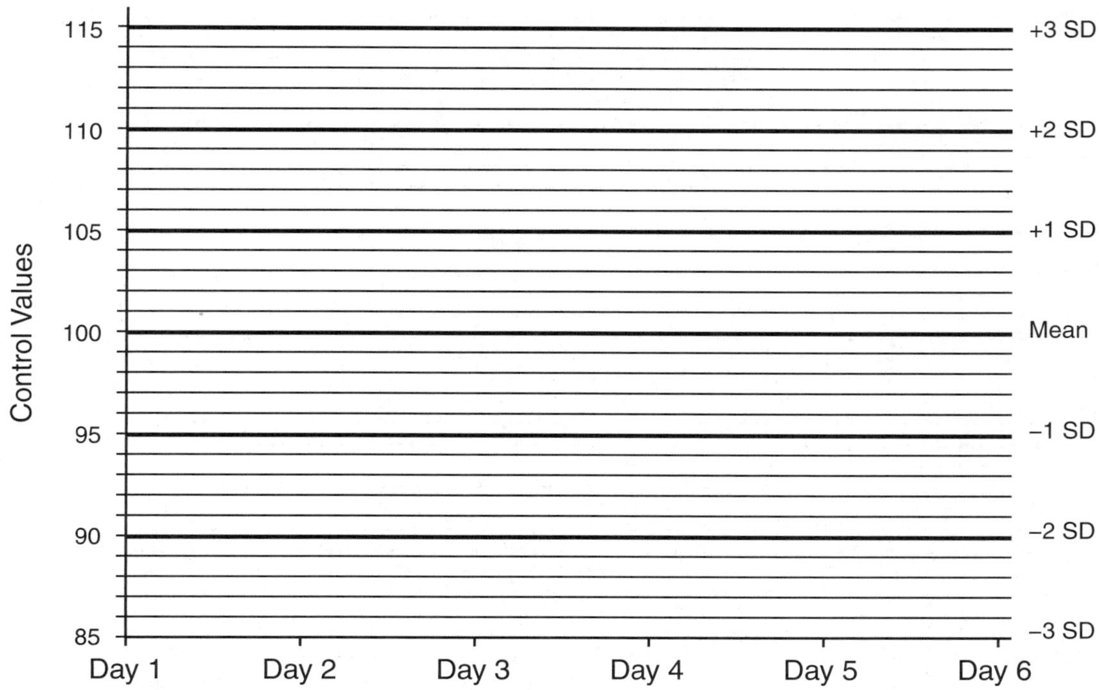

Week 2 glucose control results: ______________________

WEEK 3: day 1 = 90, day 2 = 95, day 3 = 100, day 4 = 105, day 5 = 108, day 6 = 110

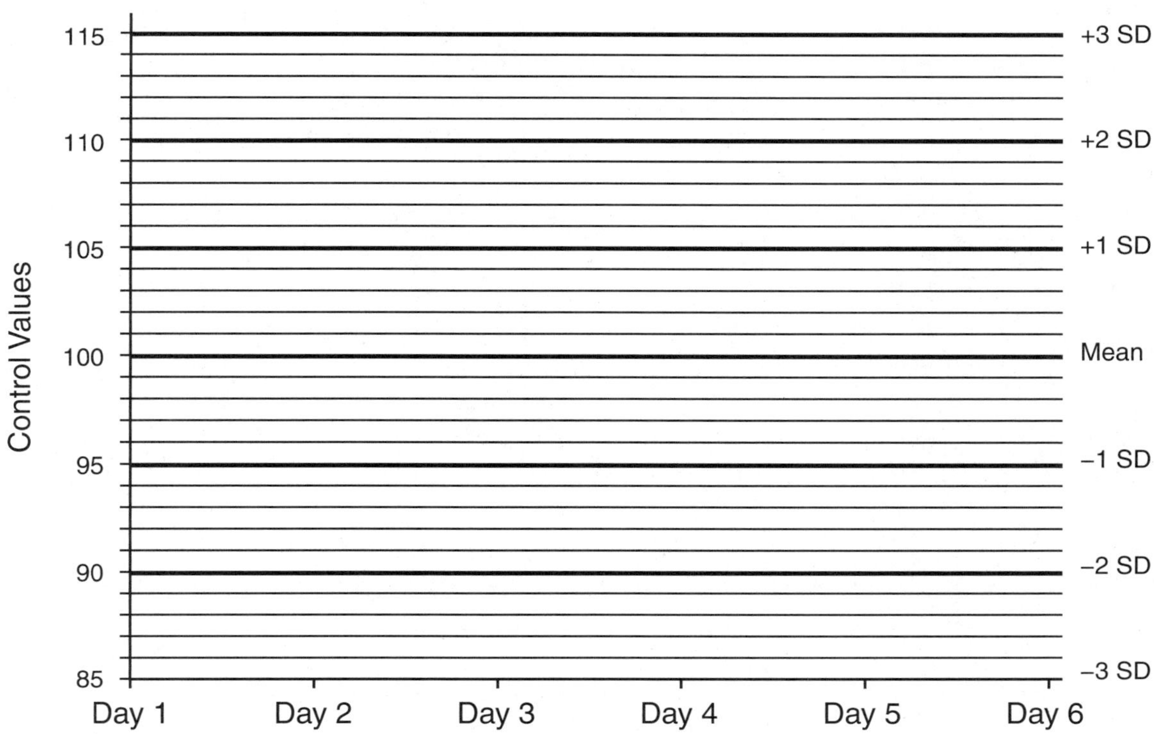

Week 3 glucose control results: ______________________

WEEK 4: day 1 = 100, day 2 = 103, day 3 = 98, day 4 = 112, day 5 = 115, day 6 = 113

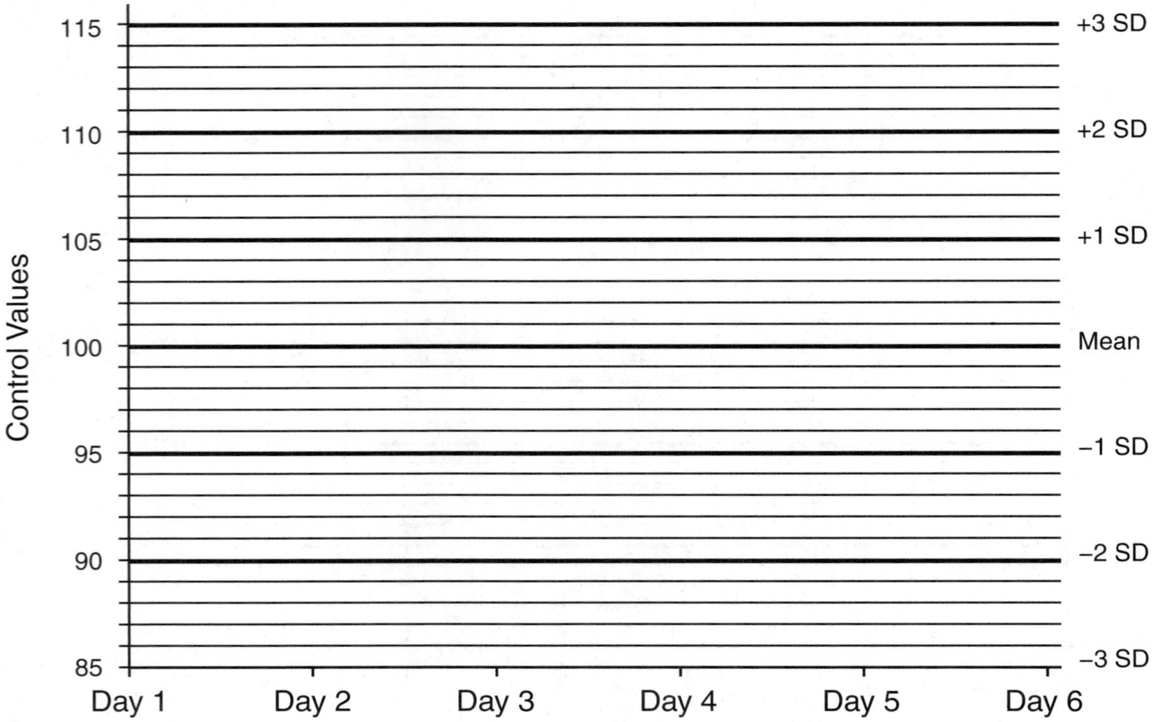

Week 4 glucose contol results: ______________________

Procedure 2-1: Using a Microscope

Person evaluated ______________________________ Date ______________

Evaluated by ______________________________ Score ______________

Outcome goal	To bring a stained slide into focus from low power to high dry power and then focus on oil immersion
Conditions	Given a microscope, lens paper, a stained slide, immersion oil, and soft, lint-free tissue
Standards	Time = 15 minutes Accuracy = each step on check sheet is completed, and an image is focused on oil immersion for evaluator check-off before cleanup
Evaluation Rubric Codes: **S** = Satisfactory, meets standard Total possible points = ____________	**U** = Unsatisfactory, fails to meet standard Points earned = ____________
NOTE: Steps marked with an asterisk (*) are critical to achieve required competency.	

Preparation	Scores	
	S	**U**
1. Carry the microscope with two hands, uncover, and adjust for cleaning.		
- Place one hand under the base, and with the other, grasp the arm of the scope.		
2. Turn the coarse focus until the stage and objectives are farthest apart.		
3. Clean the ocular and all objective lenses with lens paper (clean oil lens last).		
4. Turn the nosepiece to low power (shortest tube).		
- Do not push on objective tubes; use the nosepiece to turn.		
5. Adjust light settings.		
- Bring the condenser all the way up for a stained specimen.		
- Open the iris diaphragm all the way with the lever.		
6. Position a stained slide over the light source.		
- Place the slide with stained side up into the mechanical holder clamp.		
- By using the mechanical control, move the slide until the stained area is above the light.		
7. Adjust the ocular lens to line up with the eyes.		
Procedure	**Scores**	
	S	**U**
Low-Power Focus		
8. While looking through the oculars, turn the coarse adjustment until color starts to appear, and then turn slowly to bring the image into coarse focus.		
- Always start with the low-power objective to avoid breaking the slide.		
- Move the slide back and forth slightly with the mechanical controls to pick up movement.		

9. Move hand to fine-focus adjustment, and turn one way and then the other until the image becomes clear.		
- Make sure both eyes are seeing a clear image; if not, adjust the oculars by turning their individual focus controls.		
10. Move the slide to a place of interest in the center of the visual field, and then turn the nosepiece to high power.		
High-Power Focus		
11. Refocus the image by turning the fine adjustment one way and then the other until color is seen; then slowly bring in a clear image.		
- Do not use coarse adjustment because it will make too drastic a change and possibly break the slide. If the fine adjustment cannot focus, go back to low power, and start again with the coarse and fine-focus adjustments.		
- Move the slide so that something interesting is in the middle.		
Oil Immersion Preparation and Focus		
12. Turn the nosepiece halfway between high power and the oil immersion objective.		
13. Place a drop of oil directly on the slide where the condenser light is shining.		
14. Carefully turn the nosepiece until the oil immersion lens dips into the oil and snaps into place.		
*15. While looking into the oculars, move the small fine-focus adjustment back and forth until the image pops into view.		
*When image is in view, obtain instructor verification. ______________________		
- Scan the slide to see cells or organisms.		
- Use one hand on the mechanical control to move the slide, and use other hand on the fine focus to continuously make adjustments.		
Follow-up: Cleanup and Microscope Maintenance	**Scores**	
	S	**U**
16. Turn off the light, and turn the nosepiece back to the low-power objective.		
- Turn the coarse-focus knob to maximize the distance between the lens and stage.		
- Remove the slide, and clean the stage with soft, lint-free tissue.		
- Clean oil off the slide with the tissue or xylene.		
17. With lens paper, clean off the ocular lenses and objective lenses; the oil immersion lens is always the last to be cleaned.		
*18. Cover the microscope with a dust-proof cover, and store in a clean, protected area.		
Total Points per Column		

*The instructor or supervisor verifies a successfully focused result. This step is critical to achieve required competency.

Qualitative Test: ____________________

Person evaluated ______________________________ Date ____________________

Evaluated by ______________________________ Score ____________________

Outcome goal	
Conditions	Supplies required:
Standards	Required time = __________ minutes Performance time = __________ Total possible points = __________ Points earned = __________
Evaluation Rubric Codes: **S** = Satisfactory, meets standard **U** = Unsatisfactory, fails to meet standard	
NOTE: Steps marked with an asterisk (*) are critical to achieve required competency.	

Preparation: Preanalytical Phase	Scores	
	S	**U**
A. Test information		
- Kit method: ____________________		
- Manufacturer: ____________________		
- Proper storage (e.g., temperature, light): ____________________		
- Lot number of kit: ____________________		
- Expiration date: ____________________		
- Package insert and/or test flow chart available: __________ yes __________ no		
B. Personal protective equipment		
C. Specimen Information		

Procedure: Analytical Phase	Scores	
	S	U
D. Performed/observed qualitative quality control		
- External liquid controls: Positive ______________ Negative ______________		
- Internal control:		
E. Performed patient test		
1.		
2.		
3.		
4.		
POSITIVE seen as: NEGATIVE seen as: INVALID seen as:		
***Accurate Results** ______________ **Instructor Confirmation** ______________		

Follow-up: Postanalytical Phase	Scores	
	S	U
*F. Proper documentation		
1. On control/patient log: ______________ yes ______________ no		
2. Documented on patient chart (see below).		
3. Identified "critical values" and took appropriate steps to notify physician. **EXPECTED VALUES FOR ANALYTE:**		
G. Proper disposal and disinfection		
1. Disposed all sharps into biohazard sharps containers.		
2. Disposed all other regulated medical waste into biohazard bags.		
3. Disinfected test area and instruments according to OSHA guidelines.		
4. Sanitized hands after removing gloves.		
Total Points per Column		

Documentation on Patient Chart: Patient Name: ____

Patient Chart Entry: (Include when, what, why, any additional information, and the signature of the person charting.)

____

____

____

Analytical Testing

Quantitative Test: ______________________________

Person evaluated ______________________________ Date ______________________________

Evaluated by ______________________________ Score ______________________________

Outcome goal	
Conditions	
Standards	Required time = ____________ minutes Performance time = ____________ Total possible points = ____________ Points earned = ____________
Evaluation Rubric Codes: **S** = Satisfactory, meets standard **U** = Unsatisfactory, fails to meet standard	
NOTE: Steps marked with an asterisk (*) are critical to achieve required competency.	

Preparation: Preanalytical Phase	**Scores**	
	S	**U**
A. Test information		
- Kit or instrument method: ______________________________		
- Manufacturer: ______________________________		
- Proper storage (e.g., temperature, light): ______________________________		
- Lot number of kit or supplies: ______________________________		
- Expiration date: ______________________________		
- Package insert and/or test flow chart available: ____________ yes ____________ no		
B. Specimen Information		
- Type of specimen and its preparation (e.g., fasting, first morning): ______________________________		
- Specimen container or testing device: ______________________________		
- Amount of specimen: ______________________________		
C. Personal protective equipment		
D. Assembled all the above, sanitized hands, and applied PPE		

Procedure: Analytical Phase	Scores	
	S	U
E. Performed/observed quality control for A or B		
Quantitative testing controls		
- Calibration check: ______________		
- Control levels: Normal ______________ High ______________ Low ______________		
F. Performed patient test		
Followed proper steps (see test flow chart and list):		
1.		
2.		
3.		
4.		
5.		
6.		
7.		
8.		
9.		
10.		
***Accurate Results** ______________ **Instructor Confirmation** ______________		

Follow-up: Postanalytical Phase	Scores	
	S	U
*G. Proper documentation		
1. On control log: ______________ yes ______________ no		
2. On patient log: ______________ yes ______________ no		
3. Documented on patient chart (see next page).		
4. Identified "critical values" and took appropriate steps to notify physician.		

EXPECTED VALUES FOR ANALYTE:		
H. Proper disposal and disinfection		
1. Disposed all sharps into biohazard sharp containers.		
2. Disposed all other regulated medical waste into biohazard bags.		
3. Disinfected test area and instruments according to OSHA guidelines.		
4. Sanitized hands after removing gloves.		
Total Points per Column		

Documentation on Patient Chart: Patient Name: ______________________________

Patient Chart Entry: (Include when, what, why, any additional information, and the signature of the person charting.)

____

____

____

3 Urinalysis

VOCABULARY REVIEW

Match the function with the correct anatomic term.

_______ 1. Functional unit of the kidney

_______ 2. Part of the nephron that contains the glomerulus and glomerular capsule

_______ 3. Structure in the renal corpuscle made up of tangled blood capillaries in which the hydrostatic pressure in the capillaries pushes substances through the capillary pores

_______ 4. Cup-shaped structure surrounding the glomerulus that collects the glomerular filtrate

_______ 5. Urethral opening through which urine is expelled

_______ 6. Slender, muscular tubes 10 to 12 inches long that carry the urine formed in the kidneys to the urinary bladder

_______ 7. Hollow, muscular organ that holds urine until it is expelled

_______ 8. Tube that carries urine outside the body

_______ 9. Located behind the peritoneal cavity

_______ 10. Parts of the nephron composed of proximal convoluted tubules, the nephron loop (loop of Henle), and distal convoluted tubules

A. urethral meatus
B. glomerulus
C. glomerular capsule
D. urinary bladder
E. renal tubules
F. nephron
G. renal corpuscle
H. ureters
I. retroperitoneal
J. urethra

Match each urinalysis term with the correct definition.

_______ 11. electrolyte

_______ 12. renal threshold level

_______ 13. oliguria

_______ 14. bilirubin

_______ 15. anuria

_______ 16. dysuria

_______ 17. nocturia

_______ 18. diuresis

_______ 19. porphyrin

_______ 20. glycosuria

_______ 21. reducing substances

_______ 22. ketonuria

A. Caused by treatment or diagnostic procedures
B. Substance that easily loses electrons
C. Intact red blood cells in the urine
D. Protein found in the urine of patients with multiple myeloma
E. Painful urination
F. Red cells breaking open and releasing hemoglobin
G. Expelling of urine, also referred to as voiding and urination
H. In urinalysis, the weight of urine compared with the weight of an equal volume of water; measures the amount of dissolved substances in urine
I. No urine flow
J. Sugars (especially glucose) in the urine
K. To break open
L. Decreased urine volume
M. Ketones in the urine
N. Excessive urination at night
O. Intermediate substance in the formation of heme (part of hemoglobin)
P. Element or compound that forms ions when dissolved and is able to conduct electricity

_______ 23. hematuria

_______ 24. lyse

_______ 25. hemolysis

_______ 26. proteinuria

_______ 27. pyuria

_______ 28. iatrogenic

_______ 29. lipiduria

_______ 30. casts

_______ 31. micturition

_______ 32. pH

_______ 33. specific gravity

_______ 34. Bence Jones protein

Q. Proteins in the urine
R. Lipids in the urine
S. Increase in the volume of urine output
T. Waste product from the breakdown of hemoglobin
U. White blood cells in the urine
V. Elements excreted in the urine in the shape of the renal tubules and ducts
W. Blood reabsorption limit of a substance and the point at which the substance is then excreted in the urine
X. Scale that measures the level of acidity or alkalinity of a solution

FUNDAMENTAL CONCEPTS

Anatomy of the Urinary System

35. Label the structures of the urinary system.

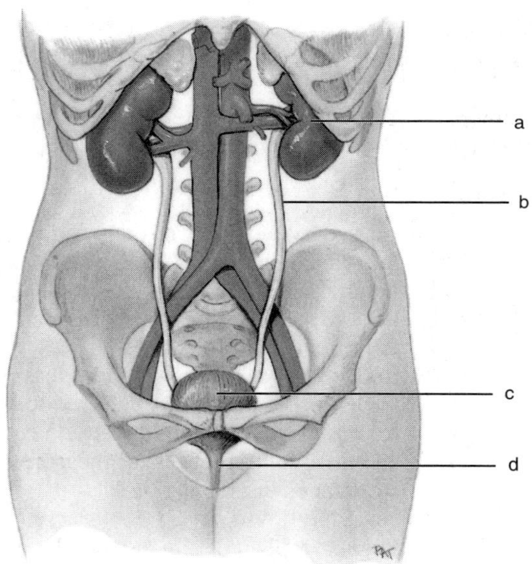

36. Label the structures of the kidney.

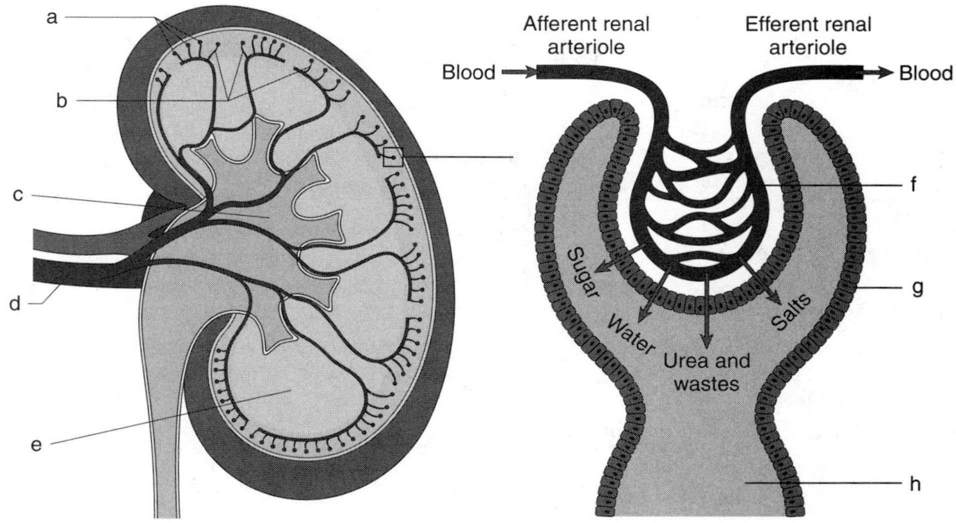

37. List three functions of the urinary system.

1. ______________________________
2. ______________________________
3. ______________________________

38. Describe the location of the kidneys in the body.

____
____

39. List the functions of the nephron.

____
____

40. Name the two structural components of the nephron.

____
____

41. List and describe the components of the renal corpuscle.

____
____
____

42. Describe the three steps of urine formation.

____
____
____

43. Explain the term *renal threshold*.

44. Discuss the importance of a urinalysis.

45. Name the three parts of a urinalysis.

Urine Specimen Collection

46. Discuss the advantages of the first morning specimen.

47. Give three general requirements for all types of urine collection methods.

48. Discuss the proper handling and discarding of urine specimens.

49. When educating a female patient about the steps involved in preparing for midstream clean catch urine, why must the patient understand the importance of wiping from front to back?

CLINICAL LABORATORY IMPROVEMENT AMENDMENT (CLIA)–WAIVED URINALYSIS TESTS

Physical Urinalysis

50. Name the tests that are part of the physical urinalysis.

51. List the terms used to describe the appearance of urine.

52. Give the range of normal color for urine.

53. In what condition can urine have a sweet or fruity odor?

54. Discuss three abnormal urine colors and their causes.

55. Describe the relevance of the specific gravity test in the urinalysis.

Chemical Urinalysis

56. Discuss the difference between qualitative, quantitative, and semiquantitative testing.

57. Label the urinalysis chemistry supplies (see Figure 3-10 in the textbook).

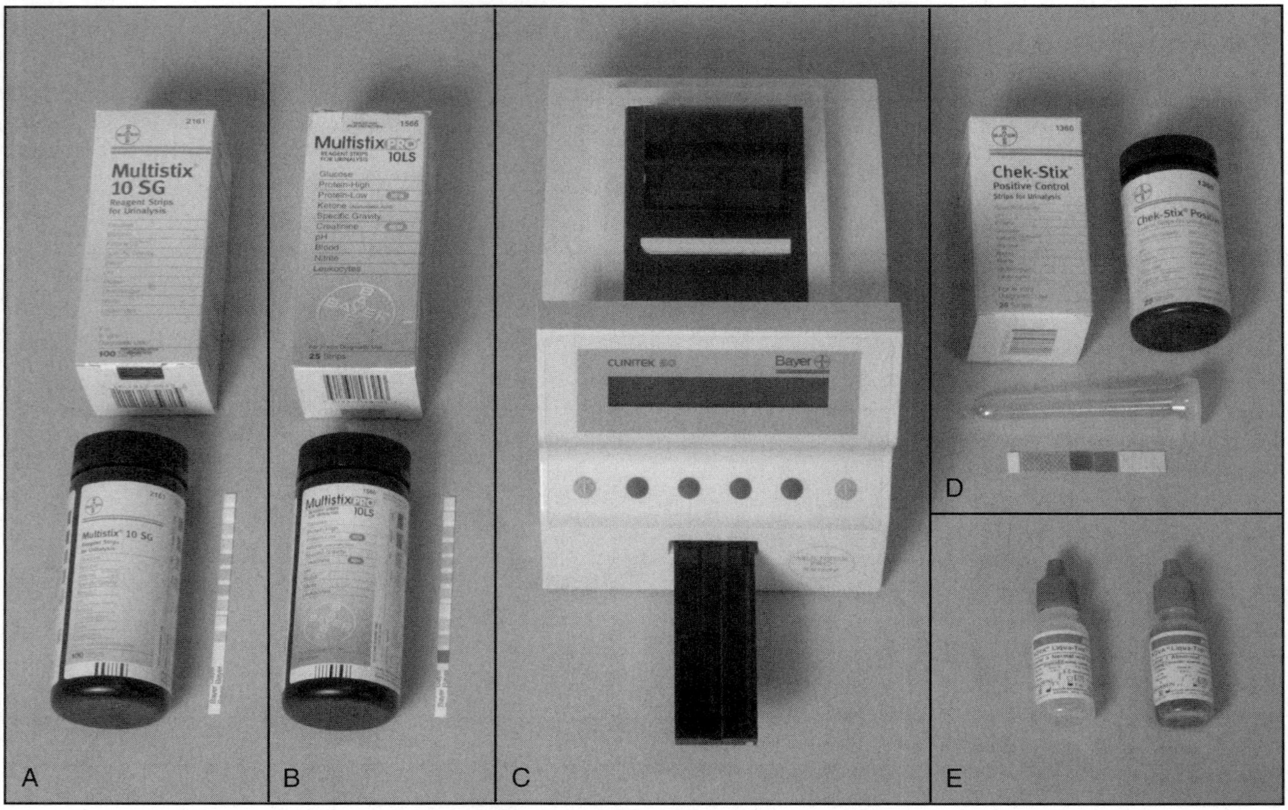

A ____________ B ____________ C ____________ D & E ____________

58. Name the 10 urinalysis chemistry tests that are most frequently performed.

1. ______________________ 6. ______________________
2. ______________________ 7. ______________________
3. ______________________ 8. ______________________
4. ______________________ 9. ______________________
5. ______________________ 10. ______________________

59. Discuss the reasons for the new method that tests for microalbumin.

____

____

____

60. List three conditions that may cause blood to be found in urine.

____

____

____

61. Explain why a first morning urine sample is recommended when testing for nitrites.

____

____

62. If the nitrite test is negative, could bacteria be present in the urine?

____

____

63. Name a confirmatory test that can be performed when a urine sample is positive for the bilirubin test.

____

64. Describe the Clinitek instrument, including its advantages and disadvantages.

____

____

____

65. List three of the urinalysis chemistry reagent strip guidelines.

____

____

____

66. Describe the quality control methods available for urinalysis chemistry testing. (Hint: see question 57.)

____

____

67. Circle the results that are abnormal compared with the urinalysis reference ranges. What is the probable cause for the abnormal urinalysis physical and chemical results, and what may the physician do next?
   - Dark yellow
   - Cloudy
   - Glucose–neg
   - Ketones–neg
   - Bilirubin–neg
   - Specific gravity 1.025
   - pH 7
   - Blood 2
   - Urobilinogen 0.2
   - Protein–mod
   - Nitrite–pos
   - Leukocyte–mod

____

____

____

68. Circle the results that are abnormal compared with the urinalysis reference ranges. What is the probable cause for the abnormal urinalysis chemical results?

- Glucose 2%
- Ketones–mod
- Bilirubin–neg
- Specific gravity 1.025
- pH 6
- Blood–neg
- Urobilinogen 0.2
- Protein–trace
- Nitrite–neg
- Leukocyte–neg

____

____

69. You just ran the Chek-Stix positive control and recorded the results shown. When looking at the expected results table for a positive control, circle the analyte that did **not** fall in its control range. Why do you suppose it did not record correctly? (Hint: Look at how the dipstick enters the urine specimen.)

Glucose–neg
Bilirubin–pos
Ketones–pos
Specific gravity 1.015
Blood large
pH 8.5
Protein 100 mg/dL
Urobilinogen 3 mg/dL
Nitrate–pos
Leukocytes–mod

	Expected Results with Bayer Reagent Strips and Tablets	
Test	**Chek-Stix Positive Control**	**Chek-Stix Negative Control**
Glucose	100-250 mg/dL	Negative
Bilirubin	Positive	Negative
Ketone	Positive	Negative
Specific gravity	1.000-1.015 (adjusted for pH)	1.010-1.025 (adjusted for pH)
Blood	Moderate, large	Negative
pH	≥8.0	6.0-7.0
Protein	Trace, 100 mg/dL (SI units: trace, 1.0 g/L)	Negative
Urobilinogen	≥2 mg/dL	0.2-1 mg/dL
Nitrite	Positive	Negative
Leukocytes	Trace, moderate	Negative
Microbumintest	Positive (by using 1:3 dilution of Chek-Stix positive control solution)	Negative
Acetest	Positive	Negative
Clinitest	250-750 mg/dL	Negative
Ictotest	Positive	Negative

70. For the standardized urinalysis Kova system for preparation of the microscopic examination, define the terms *sediment* and *supernatant,* and state which of these is used in the microscopic examination of urine.

71. List conditions in which *Candida albicans* (yeast) may be found in the urine.

72. Name the four factors that can lead to cast formation.

73. Name the crystals that resemble envelopes (with an X appearance).

74. What part of the microscopic urinalysis can be performed by a medical assistant?

75. Match the pictures of urine cells, casts, and crystals with their microscopic drawings. (See Figures 3-14 through 3-37 on pages 76 to 80 in your textbook.)

Cells

Use these terms to identify the following illustrations: Red blood cells (RBCs) on high power, squamous epithelial cells on high power, transitional epithelial cells on high power, white blood cells (WBCs) on high power.

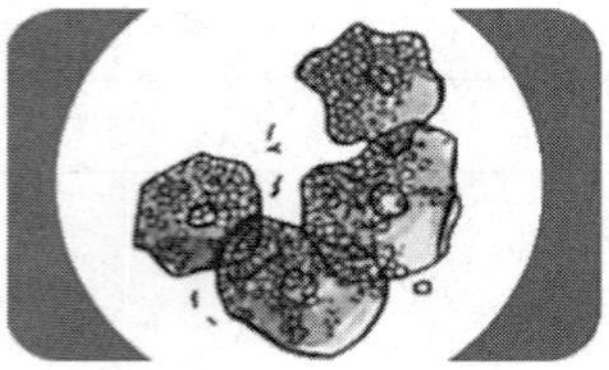

____

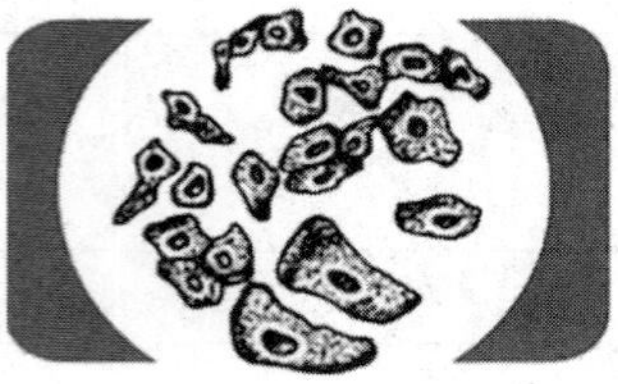

____

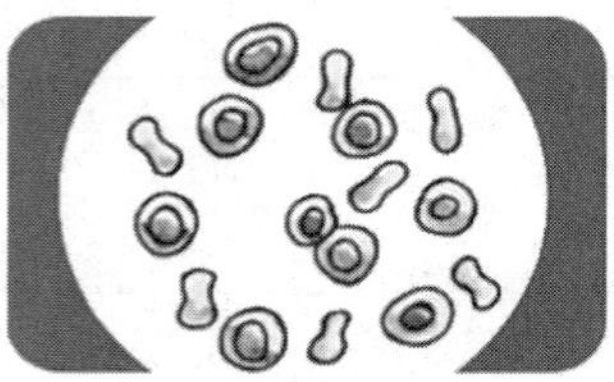

____

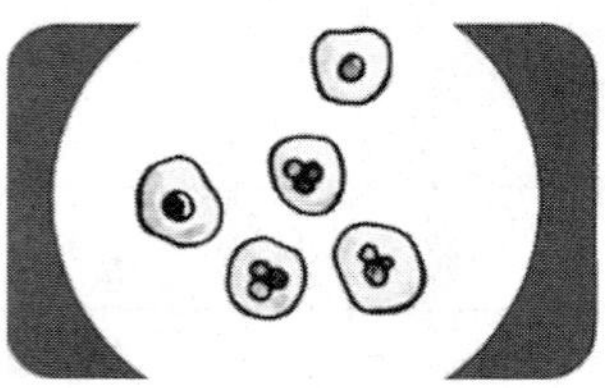

____

Casts

Use these terms to identify the following illustrations: granular casts, hyaline casts, RBC casts, WBC casts.

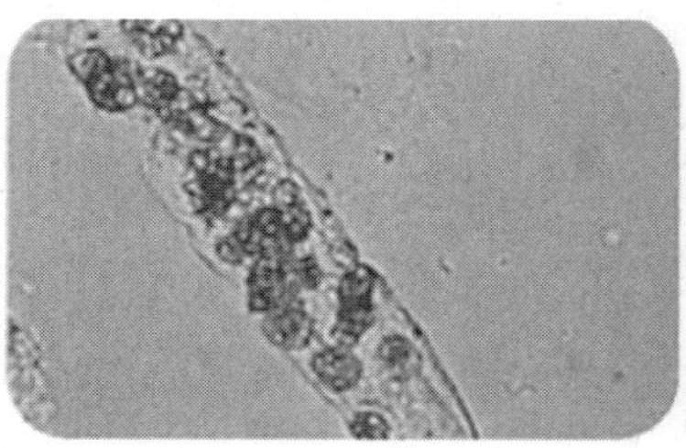

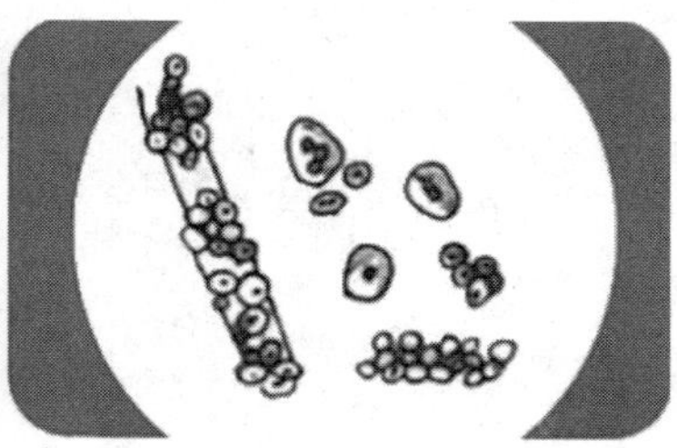

____

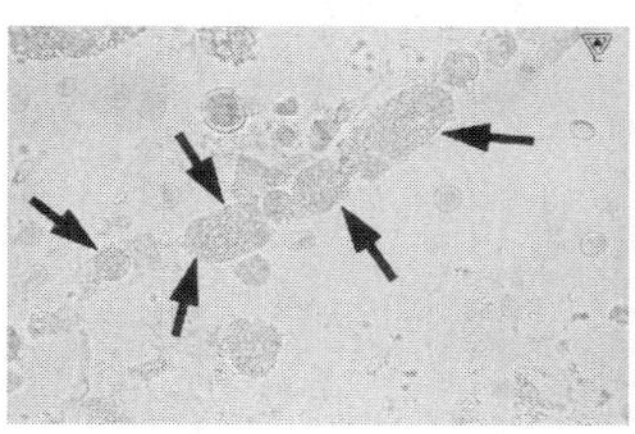

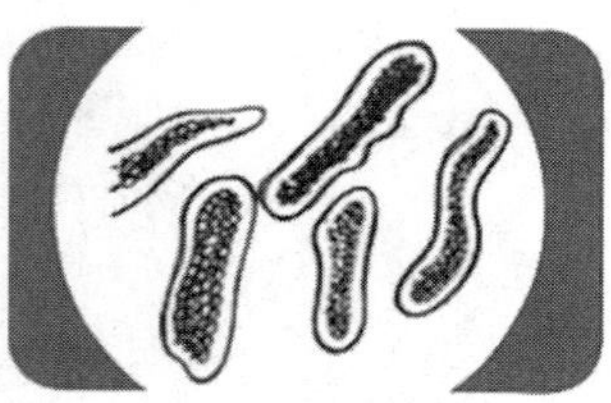

____

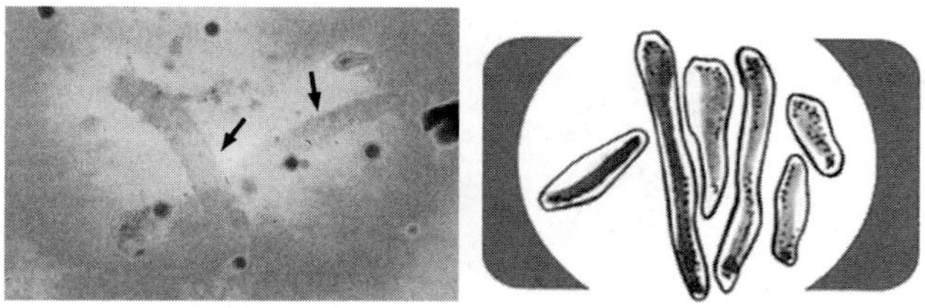

____

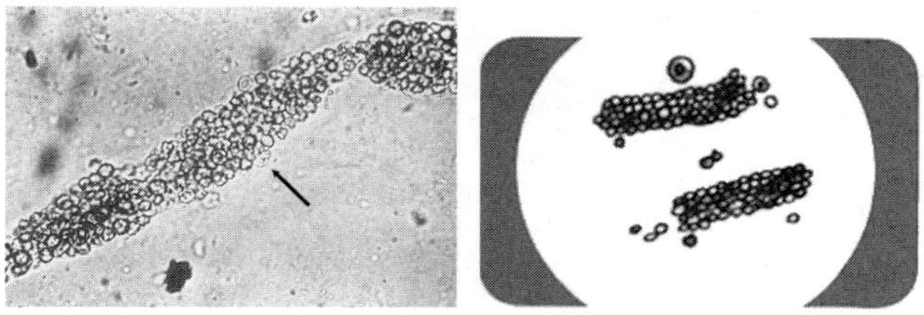

____

Crystals and Other Forms

Use these terms to identify the following illustrations: calcium oxalate crystals, *Trichomonas vaginalis*, triple phosphate crystals, yeast.

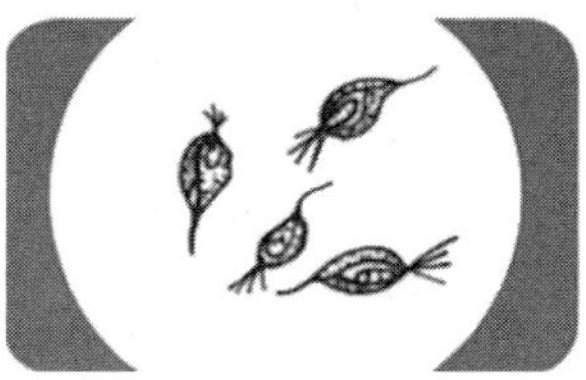

____

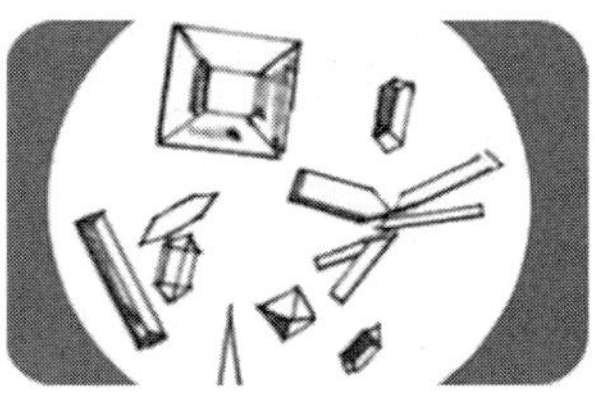

____

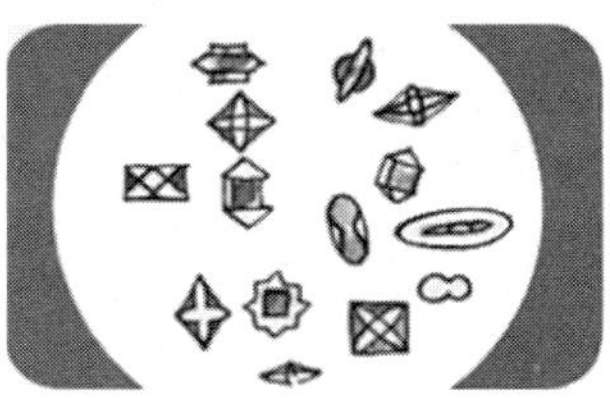

____

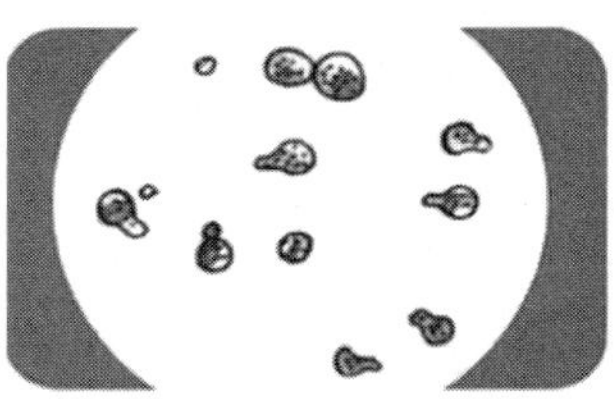

____

Procedure 3-1: Instructing Patients How to Collect a Clean-Catch Urine Specimen—Female

Person evaluated ______________________ Date______________

Evaluated by ______________________ Score______________

Outcome goal	Instruct a female patient regarding the correct procedure for midstream clean catch specimen
Conditions	Given the following: - Sterile urine collection container and label - Antiseptic towelettes
Standards	Required time = 15 minutes Performance time = __________
Evaluation Rubric Codes: **S** = Satisfactory, meets standard — **U** = Unsatisfactory, fails to meet standard Total possible points = __________ Points earned = __________	
NOTE: Steps marked with an asterisk (*) are critical to achieve required competency.	

Preparation	Scores S	Scores U
1. Washed hands and gathered the appropriate equipment.		
2. Greeted and identified the patient.		
Procedure	**S**	**U**
3. Instructed patient to sanitize her hands and remove underwear.		
4. Instructed patient to spread apart the labia to expose the urinary opening.		
- Patient told to keep this area spread apart with the nondominant hand during the entire cleaning procedure.		
5. Instructed patient to take one antiseptic towelette and clean one side of the urinary opening from front to back, stressing the importance of the direction.		
- Patient told that cleaning in this direction will prevent anal organisms from being spread to the urinary opening.		
6. Instructed patient to take another antiseptic towelette and clean other side of the urinary opening from front to back, stressing the importance of the direction.		
7. Instructed patient using a third antiseptic towelette to wipe from front to back directly across the urinary opening, stressing the importance of the direction.		
8. Instructed patient to continue to keep labia spread apart and to urinate a small amount (one third of bladder volume) into the toilet, being careful not to touch the inside of the sterile container.		
- Patient told that the reason for a small amount urinated in the toilet is to flush away microorganisms that may be around the urinary opening.		

	S	U
9. Instructed patient to collect the second part of the urine sample into the sterile container.		
- Student was able to state that this would collect the midstream portion of the urine specimen.		
10. Instructed patient to urinate the last portion of the urine into the toilet.		
11. Instructed patient to dry the area with a tissue.		
12. Instructed the patient on the correct procedure after the specimen has been collected.		
- Instructed the patient to carefully cap the specimen.		
- Instructed patient to place specimen in a certain area after collected in an office setting or to refrigerate if collected at home.		
Follow-up	**Scores**	
	S	**U**
13. After receiving the specimen from the patient, the sample was labeled correctly, and the requisition was completed if required.		
14. Washed hands.		
*15. Procedure was charted correctly.		
- Charted that female patient was given instructions for midstream clean catch urine collection.		
- Charted reception of specimen from patient.		
Total Points per Column		

Patient Chart Entry: (Include when, what, how, why, any additional information, and the signature of the person charting.)

___

___

___

Procedure 3-1: Instructing Patients How to Collect a Clean-Catch Urine Specimen—Male

Person evaluated ______________________ Date______________

Evaluated by ______________________ Score______________

Outcome goal	Instruct a male patient in the correct procedure for midstream clean catch specimen
Conditions	Given: - Sterile urine collection container and label - Antiseptic towelettes
Standards	Required time = 15 minutes Performance time = ________
Evaluation Rubric Codes: **S** = Satisfactory, meets standard Total possible points = ________	**U** = Unsatisfactory, fails to meet standard Points earned = ________
NOTE: Steps marked with an asterisk (*) are critical to achieve required competency.	

Preparation	**Scores S**	**Scores U**
1. Washed hands and gathered the appropriate equipment.		
2. Greeted and identified the patient.		
Procedure	**S**	**U**
3. Instructed patient to sanitize his hands and remove underwear.		
4. If patient is uncircumcised, instructed the patient to retract the foreskin and hold it back during the entire procedure.		
5. Instructed the patient to clean the area around the penis opening by starting at the tip of the penis and cleaning downward, using a separate antiseptic towelette for each side.		
6. Instructed patient to use a third antiseptic towelette to clean across the opening.		
*7. Instructed patient to urinate a small amount (one third of bladder volume) into the toilet, being careful not to touch the inside of the sterile container.		
- Patient told that the reason for a small amount urinated in the toilet is to flush away microorganisms that may be around the urinary opening.		
8. Instructed patient to collect the second part of the urine sample into the sterile container.		
- Student was able to state that this would collect the midstream portion of the urine specimen.		
9. Instructed patient to urinate the last portion of the urine into the toilet.		
10. Instructed patient to dry the area with a tissue if needed.		

Follow-up	Scores	
	S	U
11. Instructed the patient on the correct procedure after the specimen has been collected.		
- Instructed the patient to carefully cap the specimen.		
- Instructed patient to place specimen in a certain area after collected in an office setting or to refrigerate if collected at home.		
12. After receiving the specimen from the patient, the sample was labeled correctly and the requisition was completed if required.		
13. Washed hands.		
*14. Charted procedure correctly.		
- Charted that male patient was given instructions for midstream clean catch urine collection.		
- Charted reception of specimen from patient.		
Total Points per Column		

Patient Chart Entry: (Include when, what, how, why, any additional information, and the signature of the person charting.)

____

____

____

Procedure 3-2: Instructing Patients How to Collect a 24-Hour Urine Specimen

Person evaluated ______________________ Date______________

Evaluated by ______________________ Score______________

Outcome goal	To educate the patient on the correct instructions for collection of a 24-hour urine specimen
Conditions	Given: - Large urine container - Instructions sheet - Requisition
Standards	Required time = 15 minutes Performance time = __________
Evaluation Rubric Codes: **S** = Satisfactory, meets standard **U** = Unsatisfactory, fails to meet standard Total possible points = __________ Points earned = __________	
NOTE: Steps marked with an asterisk (*) are critical to achieve required competency.	

Preparation	Scores	
	S	**U**
1. Washed hands and gathered the appropriate equipment.		
2. Greeted and identified the patient.		
Procedure	**Scores**	
	S	**U**
3. Instructed patient when arising on the first day of the 24-hour collection procedure to empty bladder into the toilet.		
- Instructed patient to record this time.		
4. Instructed the patient that all urine for 24 hours after that first voided specimen must be voided directly into the collection container.		
- Informed the patient to be sure to screw the lid on tightly each time and keep the container refrigerated.		
- Informed the patient that if at any time during the procedure some urine is not collected, the test will need to start again. Gave examples of this.		
5. Instructed the patient that on the second morning of the 24-hour period the patient must arise at the same time as the first day and urinate directly into the container, keeping this sample.		
- Patient was instructed that the first morning specimen on the second day 24-hour period is the last sample collected and is the completion of the collection procedure.		
6. Instructed the patient that on the day the procedure is completed, the container must be returned to the physician's office or to the laboratory.		

Follow-up	Scores	
	S	U
7. After the patient completed the procedure and returned the container, the patient was asked if any problems occurred during the collection procedure.		
8. Completed a laboratory requisition form for test ordered.		
9. Prepared the specimen to be transported to the laboratory that will perform the testing.		
*10. Charted the instructions and equipment supplied to the patient.		
- When patient returned with specimen, charted that the specimen was sent to the laboratory, documenting all necessary information concerning the specimen.		
Total Points per Column		

Patient Chart Entry: (Include when, what, how, why, any additional information, and the signature of the person charting.)

____

____

____

Procedure 3-3: Manual Chemical Reagent Strip Procedure

Person evaluated ________________________________ Date______________________

Evaluated by ________________________________ Score______________________

Outcome goal	Perform a physical and chemical test on an unknown sample according to stated conditions and standards
Conditions	Given: - Reagent strips - Timing device - Reference chart - Requisition
Standards	Required time = 10 minutes Performance time = ____________
Evaluation Rubric Codes: **S** = Satisfactory, meets standard Total possible points = ____________	**U** = Unsatisfactory, fails to meet standard Points earned = ____________

Preparation: Preanalytical Phase	Scores	
	S	**U**
A. Test information		
- Kit or instrument method: **Multistix 10 SG**		
- Manufacturer: **Bayer Corporation**		
- Proper storage (e.g., temperature, light): **room temperature, no direct sunlight**		
- Expiration date: ____________		
- Lot number: ____________		
- Package insert or test flow chart: _____ yes _____ no		
B. Proper specimen		
- Special patient preparation (e.g., fasting, special diet, first morning specimen): **no special preparation**		
- Appropriate container: **clean container without preservatives**		
- Amount of specimen: **25 to 50 mL well-mixed urine**		
C. Personal protective equipment: **gloves, gown, and biohazard container**		
Procedure: Analytical Phase	**Scores**	
	S	**U**
*D. Performed/observed quality control methods		
1. Semiquantitative liquid controls		
- Control levels: Normal ____________ Abnormal ____________		

*E. Performed patient test	S	U
1. Hands were sanitized and equipment assembled.		
2. Urine was poured into a clear container or centrifuge tube.		
3. The color of the urine was determined.		
4. The clarity of the urine was determined.		
5. Strip was removed from the bottle, and the bottle was immediately closed. The pads on the strip were not touched, and the strip was held parallel to the chart.		
6. The pads were completely covered with urine. The pads were not immersed too long, which could cause the reagents to dissolve and leach out into the urine.		
7. After removing the strip from the urine, the strip was tapped against the side of the tube to remove excess urine.		
8. The color of each strip pad was read at a particular time and compared with the reference chart.		
***Accurate Results (see attached forms) Instructor Confirmation** ___________		

Follow-up: Postanalytical Phase	**Scores**	
	S	**U**
*F. Proper documentation: ___________		
1. On control log: ___________ yes ___________ no		
2. On patient log: ___________ yes ___________ no		
3. Documentation on patient chart forms on next page.		
4. Identified critical values and took appropriate steps to notify physician.		

Analyte Expected Values

Glucose	**Neg**
Bilirubin	**Neg**
Ketone	**Neg**
Specific gravity	**1.005-1.030**
Blood	**Neg**
pH	**6.0-8.0**
Protein	**Neg/trace**
Urobilirubin	**Norm**
Nitrite	**Neg**
Leukocytes	**Neg**

G. Proper disposal and disinfection		
1. Disposed strip into appropriate biohazard containers.		
2. Poured the remaining urine down sink with stream of water and placed container in appropriate waste container.		
3. Disinfected test area and instruments according to OSHA guidelines.		
4. Sanitized hands after removing gloves.		
Total Points per Column		

Patient: Date/Time Spec. Collected:

Doctor: DOB: Date/Time Spec. Completed:

	TEST	REFERENCE	RESULT	TEST	REFERENCE	RESULT		TEST	REFERENCE	RESULT	TEST	REFERENCE	RESULT
☐ VOID	Color	Yellow		Blood	Neg		MICRO	WBC	0 - 5 HPF		Bact.	0 - 5	
☐ CC	Char.	Clear		pH	5.0 - 8.0			RBC	0 - 3 HPF		Mucus	0	
☐ CATH	Glucose	Neg		Protein	Neg			Epith.	D		Casts	0	
☐ TURBID	Bilirubin	Neg		Urobili	0.2 - 1.0 EU			Cryst.	0 - 3 HPF				
☐ HAZY	Ketone	Neg		Nitrite	Neg		OTHER:						
☐ CLEAR	Sp. Gr	1,000-1,030		Leuk	Neg								

Patient: Date/Time Spec. Collected:

Doctor: DOB: Date/Time Spec. Completed:

	TEST	REFERENCE	RESULT	TEST	REFERENCE	RESULT		TEST	REFERENCE	RESULT	TEST	REFERENCE	RESULT
☐ VOID	Color	Yellow		Blood	Neg		MICRO	WBC	0 - 5 HPF		Bact.	0 - 5	
☐ CC	Char.	Clear		pH	5.0 - 8.0			RBC	0 - 3 HPF		Mucus	0	
☐ CATH	Glucose	Neg		Protein	Neg			Epith.	D		Casts	0	
☐ TURBID	Bilirubin	Neg		Urobili	0.2 - 1.0 EU			Cryst.	0 - 3 HPF				
☐ HAZY	Ketone	Neg		Nitrite	Neg		OTHER:						
☐ CLEAR	Sp. Gr	1,000-1,030		Leuk	Neg								

Patient: Date/Time Spec. Collected:

Doctor: DOB: Date/Time Spec. Completed:

	TEST	REFERENCE	RESULT	TEST	REFERENCE	RESULT		TEST	REFERENCE	RESULT	TEST	REFERENCE	RESULT
☐ VOID	Color	Yellow		Blood	Neg		MICRO	WBC	0 - 5 HPF		Bact.	0 - 5	
☐ CC	Char.	Clear		pH	5.0 - 8.0			RBC	0 - 3 HPF		Mucus	0	
☐ CATH	Glucose	Neg		Protein	Neg			Epith.	D		Casts	0	
☐ TURBID	Bilirubin	Neg		Urobili	0.2 - 1.0 EU			Cryst.	0 - 3 HPF				
☐ HAZY	Ketone	Neg		Nitrite	Neg		OTHER:						
☐ CLEAR	Sp. Gr	1,000-1,030		Leuk	Neg								

Patient: Date/Time Spec. Collected:

Doctor: DOB: Date/Time Spec. Completed:

	TEST	REFERENCE	RESULT	TEST	REFERENCE	RESULT		TEST	REFERENCE	RESULT	TEST	REFERENCE	RESULT
☐ VOID	Color	Yellow		Blood	Neg		MICRO	WBC	0 - 5 HPF		Bact.	0 - 5	
☐ CC	Char.	Clear		pH	5.0 - 8.0			RBC	0 - 3 HPF		Mucus	0	
☐ CATH	Glucose	Neg		Protein	Neg			Epith.	D		Casts	0	
☐ TURBID	Bilirubin	Neg		Urobili	0.2 - 1.0 EU			Cryst.	0 - 3 HPF				
☐ HAZY	Ketone	Neg		Nitrite	Neg		OTHER:						
☐ CLEAR	Sp. Gr	1,000-1,030		Leuk	Neg								

Patient: Date/Time Spec. Collected:

Doctor: DOB: Date/Time Spec. Completed:

	TEST	REFERENCE	RESULT	TEST	REFERENCE	RESULT		TEST	REFERENCE	RESULT	TEST	REFERENCE	RESULT
☐ VOID	Color	Yellow		Blood	Neg		MICRO	WBC	0 - 5 HPF		Bact.	0 - 5	
☐ CC	Char.	Clear		pH	5.0 - 8.0			RBC	0 - 3 HPF		Mucus	0	
☐ CATH	Glucose	Neg		Protein	Neg			Epith.	D		Casts	0	
☐ TURBID	Bilirubin	Neg		Urobili	0.2 - 1.0 EU			Cryst.	0 - 3 HPF				
☐ HAZY	Ketone	Neg		Nitrite	Neg		OTHER:						
☐ CLEAR	Sp. Gr	1,000-1,030		Leuk	Neg								

Patient: Date/Time Spec. Collected:

Doctor: DOB: Date/Time Spec. Completed:

	TEST	REFERENCE	RESULT	TEST	REFERENCE	RESULT		TEST	REFERENCE	RESULT	TEST	REFERENCE	RESULT
☐ VOID	Color	Yellow		Blood	Neg		MICRO	WBC	0 - 5 HPF		Bact.	0 - 5	
☐ CC	Char.	Clear		pH	5.0 - 8.0			RBC	0 - 3 HPF		Mucus	0	
☐ CATH	Glucose	Neg		Protein	Neg			Epith.	D		Casts	0	
☐ TURBID	Bilirubin	Neg		Urobili	0.2 - 1.0 EU			Cryst.	0 - 3 HPF				
☐ HAZY	Ketone	Neg		Nitrite	Neg		OTHER:						
☐ CLEAR	Sp. Gr	1,000-1,030		Leuk	Neg								

Procedure 3-4: Clinitek Analyzer Method for Chemical Reagent Strip

Person evaluated ______________________ Date______________

Evaluated by ______________________ Score______________

Outcome goal	Perform a physical and chemical test on an unknown sample according to stated conditions and standards
Conditions	Given: - Gloves - Multistix 10SG reagent strips or MultistixPro10SL strips - Absorbent paper - Clinitek analyzer
Standards	Required time = 5 minutes Performance time = ____________
Evaluation Rubric Codes: **S** = Satisfactory, meets standard Total possible points = ____________	**U** = Unsatisfactory, fails to meet standard Points earned = ____________

Preparation: Preanalytical Phase	**Scores**	
	S	**U**
A. Test information		
- Kit or instrument method: **Multistix 10 SG and Clinitek instrument**		
- Manufacturer: **Bayer Corporation**		
- Proper storage (e.g., temperature, light): **room temperature, no direct sunlight**		
- Expiration date: ____________		
- Lot number: ______________		
- Package insert or test flow chart: _____ yes _____ no		
B. Proper specimen		
- Special patient preparation (e.g., fasting, special diet, first morning specimen): **no special preparation**		
- Appropriate container: **clean container without preservatives**		
- Amount of specimen: **25 to 50 mL well-mixed urine**		
C. Personal protective equipment: **gloves, gown, and biohazard container**		

Procedure: Analytical Phase	Scores	
	S	U
*D. Performed/observed quality control methods		
1. Semiquantitative liquid controls		
- Control levels: Normal (negative) ____________ Abnormal (positive) ____________		
*E. Performed patient test	S	U
1. Mixed the room-temperature urine sample, and poured it into a conical tube before testing.		
2. Removed the strip from the bottle, closed it immediately. Did not touch the reagent pads.		
3. Followed the instructions on the instrument monitor or the manufacturer's flow sheet. • Entered technician identification. • Entered patient information. • Before pressing the "start" command, had test strip ready to dip into the urine.		
4. After pressing start, completed the following within 8 seconds. • **Dipped** the strip into the urine, making sure all the pads were completely covered with urine, but did not immerse it too long. • **Removed** excess urine from the strip by pulling the nonpad side of the strip along the edge of the container. • **Blotted** the side of the strip against absorbent paper briefly. • **Placed** the strip in the Clinitek tray, making sure it was placed correctly.		
5. *Note:* If the reagent strip was placed incorrectly, an error message appeared, and the tray pushed the sample out. The reagent strip was discarded, the instrument was reset, and a new reagent strip was used to run the test again.		
6. While the instrument was measuring timed reagent pads, recorded the color and transparency of the urine specimen.		
7. When the test was complete, the analyzer displayed and printed the date, the time, the patient's name, the name of the person testing, the results of the 10 tests, the color, and a transparency.		
***Accurate Results (see attached forms or printed form) Instructor Confirmation** ________		

Follow-up: Postanalytical Phase	Scores	
	S	U
*F. Proper documentation ____________		
1. On control log: ____________ yes ____________ no		
2. On patient log: ____________ yes ____________ no		
3. Documentation on patient chart forms on previous pages.		

4. Identified critical values and took appropriate steps to notify physician.		

Analyte Expected Values

Glucose	**Neg**
Bilirubin	**Neg**
Ketone	**Neg**
Specific gravity	**1.005-1.030**
Blood	**Neg**
pH	**6.0-8.0**
Protein	**Neg/trace**
Urobilirubin	**Norm**
Nitrite	**Neg**
Leukocytes	**Neg**

G. Proper disposal and disinfection		
1. Disposed strip into appropriate biohazard containers.		
2. Disposed all other regulated medical waste into biohazard bags.		
3. Disinfected test area and instruments according to OSHA guidelines.		
4. Sanitized hands after removing gloves.		
Total Points per Column		

Procedure 3-5: Clinitest Procedure for Reducing Substances Such as Sugars in the Urine

Person evaluated ______________________ Date ______________

Evaluated by ______________________ Score ______________

Outcome goal	Perform a Clinitest test on an unknown sample
Conditions	Given: - Clinitest bottle of tablets - Clinitest tube - Tube of water with pipette - Urine sample with pipette - Clinitest reference chart
Standards	Required time = 5 minutes Performance time = ______
Evaluation Rubric Codes: **S** = Satisfactory, meets standard Total possible points = ______	**U** = Unsatisfactory, fails to meet standard Points earned = ______
NOTE: Steps marked with an asterisk (*) are critical to achieve required competency	

Preparation: Preanalytical Phase	**Scores S**	**Scores U**
A. Test information		
- Kit or instrument method: **Clinitest**		
- Manufacturer: **Bayer Corporation**		
- Proper storage (e.g., temperature, light): **room temperature with the lid tightly sealed; protect tablets from light, heat, and moisture**		
- Lot number of kit: ______		
- Expiration date: ______		
- Package insert available: ______ yes ______ no		
B. Specimen information		
- Labeled urine specimen in clean container		
- Amount: **2 or 5 drops (according to directions)**		
C. Personal protective equipment: **gloves, sharps, and biohazard**		

Procedure: Analytical Phase	Scores S	Scores U
D. Performed/observed quality control		
1. Semiquantitative testing controls		
- Control levels: Normal ____________ Abnormal ____________		
E. Performed patient test	S	U
1. Added 5 drops of urine to 10 drops of water in a Clinitest tube.		
2. Tapped the Clinitest tablet into the tube, which was placed in a rack because the boiling reaction that occurs is very hot.		
3. During the boiling reaction, the tube was observed for any color change.		
- The boiling reaction should be observed for the "pass through effect," which results with color change occurring during the reaction and appears negative when the reaction is completed and results are determined.		
4. Shook the tube 15 seconds after the boiling had stopped to mix the contents.		
5. Compared color of the reaction with the Clinitest chart for the 5-drop method and recorded the results.		
***Accurate Results ____________ Instructor Confirmation ____________**		

Follow-up: Postanalytical Phase	Scores S	Scores U
*F. Proper documentation____________		
1. On control log: ____________ yes ____________ no		
2. On patient log: ____________ yes ____________ no		
3. Documentation on patient chart (see below).		
4. Identified critical values and took appropriate steps to notify physician. Expected values for analyte: **negative**		
G. Proper disposal and disinfection		
1. Disposed all other regulated medical waste into biohazard bags.		
2. Disinfected test area and instruments according to OSHA guidelines.		
3. Sanitized hands after removing gloves.		
Total Points per Column		

Patient Name: ____

Patient Chart Entry: (Include when, how, what, why, any additional information, and the signature of the person charting.)

____

____

____

Procedure 3-6: Procedure for the Preparation and the Microscopic Examination of Urine

Person evaluated ______________________ Date______________

Evaluated by ______________________ Score______________

Outcome goal	To prepare a microscopic urinalysis slide, focus the slide on the microscope, and state the elements that can be found under low and high power
Conditions	Given: - Gloves - Urine specimen - Kova equipment: cap, pipette - Sternheimer-Malbin stain - Test tube - Centrifuge - Microscope
Standards	Required time = 5 minutes Performance time = __________
Evaluation Rubric Codes: **S** = Satisfactory, meets standard Total possible points = __________	**U** = Unsatisfactory, fails to meet standard Points earned = __________
NOTE: Steps marked with an asterisk (*) are critical to achieve required competency.	

Preparation	Scores	
	S	**U**
1. Washed hands, applied gloves, and gathered the appropriate equipment.		
2. Mixed the correctly identified room temperature urine specimen.		
3. Poured the urine sample to the "12 mark" in a urine centrifuge tube and capped the tube.		
Procedure	**Scores**	
	S	**U**
4. Centrifuged the tube for 5 minutes at 1500 rpm.		
- Stated the definition of sediment and supernatant.		
5. Carefully removed the spun tube from the centrifuge and removed the cap.		
6. Carefully placed the Kova pipette into the bottom of the tube.		
- Hooked the clip on the top of the pipette over the outside of the tube.		
7. Placed index finger on tip of the pipette and decanted off the supernatant by inverting the tube.		
- Stated the approximate amount of sediment that remained in the tube.		

	S	U
8. Removed the pipette from the tube, added a drop of stain, and reinserted the pipette, squeezing gently to mix the urine sediment and stain.		
- Stated the purpose of using the stain.		
9. Correctly transferred a drop of the urine sediment to a well in a Kova slide.		
- Did not overfill or underfill the well.		
10. Allowed the Kova slide to sit for 1 minute.		
- Stated why the slide should sit.		
11. Stated who is qualified to perform a urine microscopic examination.		
12. Demonstrated the ability to focus a slide on the microscope.		
- Focused first with low power with the course adjustment.		
- Was able to fine focus with the fine adjustment knob.		
*13. Stated what elements are observed under low power.		
*14. Stated what elements are observed under high power.		
***Accurate Results** ______ **Instructor Confirmation** ______		
Follow-up: Postanalytical Phase	**Scores**	
	S	**U**
15. Demonstrated the proper procedure for cleaning, carrying, and storing the microscope.		
16. Correctly discarded the equipment in the appropriate containers.		
- Discarded the urine specimen in the appropriate manner.		
17. Removed and discarded gloves in the appropriate biohazard containers.		
18. Sanitized hands.		
19. Demonstrated an understanding of the process for calculating a urinalysis microscopic examination.		
Total Points per Column		

Patient Chart Entry: (Include when, what, how, why, any additional information, and the signature of the person charting.)

____

____

____

4 Blood Collection

VOCABULARY REVIEW

Match each term with the correct definition.

_______ 1. cyanotic
_______ 2. edema
_______ 3. syncope
_______ 4. petechiae
_______ 5. plasma
_______ 6. veins
_______ 7. antecubital space
_______ 8. capillary action
_______ 9. arteries
_______ 10. hematoma
_______ 11. interstitial fluid
_______ 12. phlebotomy
_______ 13. serum
_______ 14. osteomyelitis
_______ 15. capillaries
_______ 16. buffy coat
_______ 17. humors
_______ 18. evacuate
_______ 19. palpating
_______ 20. hemoconcentration
_______ 21. lumen
_______ 22. microcollection

A. Area in front of the elbow
B. Blood vessels that carry blood away from the heart
C. Microscopic blood vessels that contain a mixture of arterial and venous blood
D. Process by which blood flows freely into a capillary tube in microcollection procedures
E. Condition in which the skin and mucous membranes are blue; caused by an oxygen deficiency
F. Abnormal collection of fluid in interstitial spaces
G. Tumor or swelling of blood in the tissues (resulting in bruising during blood collection procedures)
H. All the fluid, except blood, found in the space between tissues; also referred to as tissue fluid
I. Inflammation of the bone caused by bacterial infection
J. Tiny purple or red skin spots caused by small amounts of blood under the skin; found in those with coagulation problems; can lead to excessive bleeding during phlebotomy procedures
K. Blood collection; derived from the Greek words *phlebo,* meaning vein, and *tomy,* meaning to cut
L. Liquid part of whole blood
M. Liquid part obtained when blood is clotted; lacks the clotting factors
N. Blood vessels that carry blood toward the heart
O. Fainting
P. Gently touching and pressing down on an area to feel texture, size, and consistency
Q. Narrow middle layer of white blood cells and platelets in a centrifuged whole blood specimen
R. Fluid or semifluid substances found in the body
S. Inner tubular space of a needle, vessel, or tube
T. Condition in which blood concentration of large molecules such as proteins, cells, and coagulation factors increases
U. Collecting a small amount of blood
V. Removing air to produce a vacuum

FUNDAMENTAL CONCEPTS

23. Explain the differences between arteries, arterioles, capillaries, venules, and veins.

____
____
____
____

24. Determine if the following substances are higher in the capillary or venous blood.

a. Hemoglobin ______________________

b. Total protein ______________________

c. Potassium ______________________

d. Glucose ______________________

e. Calcium ______________________

25. Describe the difference in the "feel" between an artery and a vein.

____

____

26. Draw a diagram of the most common veins in the antecubital area used for phlebotomy.

27. List the seven items that must be on a requisition.

a. ______________________

b. ______________________

c. ______________________

d. ______________________

e. ______________________

f. ______________________

g. ______________________

28. What is the most critical error that a phlebotomist can make?

____

____

29. Describe the three-way match for patient identification.

____

____

30. Explain the proper way to determine a patient's name.

____

____

31. Describe and explain the correct positions of a patient when performing phlebotomy.

____

____

BLOOD COLLECTION PROCEDURES

Capillary Puncture

32. Describe the composition of capillary blood.

____

____

____

33. Label the capillary puncture supplies.

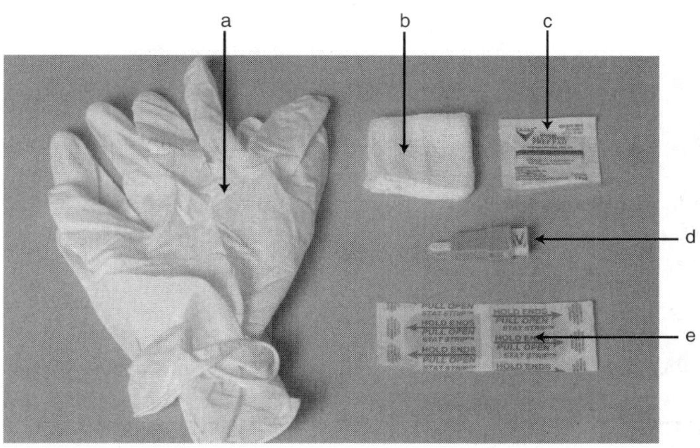

34. List three situations when capillary blood may be used and three situations when this method should not be used.

____

____

____

____

____

____

35. What is the recommended capillary puncture depth for newborns and infants? Explain why.

____

____

36. List two types of tubes that can be used to collect the blood from capillary punctures. (Hint: see Figure 4-6C and D in the textbook.)

____

____

37. List and explain the recommended order of collecting the various colored microtainers from a capillary puncture.

____

____

____

____

38. Describe the appropriate capillary puncture collection sites for adults and children and then for newborns and infants.

Adults and children: _______________

____

Infants and newborns: _______________

____

39. Why is the first drop of blood wiped away in a capillary puncture?

____

____

40. Discuss the effects if alcohol is not allowed to dry when performing blood collection.

____

____

41. What will squeezing the puncture site do to the test results?

____

____

42. Describe what to do if the blood stops flowing and not enough blood was obtained.

____

____

43. Describe phenylketonuria (PKU).

____

____

44. Describe the neonatal screening collection procedure.

____

____

____

____

45. Discuss the infant age parameters for testing for PKU.

____

____

46. In the following case study steps, write **C** if the technique is correct or **I** if the technique is incorrect; explain why in the space provided.
A medical assistant performs a capillary puncture on an adult.

_______ 1. The medical assistant washes his or her hands and puts on gloves.

____

_______ 2. The site that is chosen is the lateral part of the fingertip (slightly to the side of center) of the middle finger.

____

_______ 3. The site is cleaned with 30% alcohol.

____

_______ 4. The puncture is made before the site is dry.

____

_______ 5. The puncture is made parallel to the whorls of the fingerprint.

____

47. In the following scenario about a capillary puncture, circle the incorrect techniques. In the space provided, explain the repercussions that could occur from using the incorrect method.

A capillary puncture is performed on the central area of the heel of a newborn infant's foot. The area is cleaned with 70% alcohol, and before it has dried, a puncture is made with a lancet to a depth of 3 mm. Immediately after the puncture, the blood is collected in a capillary tube by squeezing the puncture site. After all the blood has been obtained, pressure is applied to the puncture site, and an adhesive bandage is applied.

____

____

____

____

____

48. Explain the difference between serum and plasma, and describe how each is obtained.

____

____

49. Label the parts of the Vacutainer system.

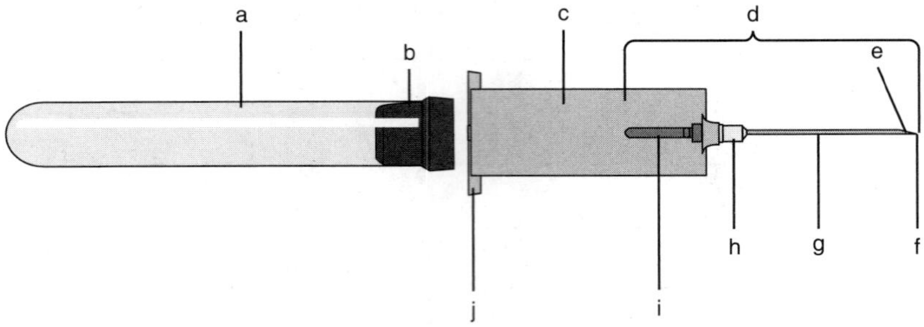

50. Place the following tubes in the correct order of draw, and name the anticoagulant or additive in each: green, gray, red, lavender.

a. ______________________; ______________________

b. ______________________; ______________________

c. ______________________; ______________________

d. ______________________; ______________________

51. Describe how a gel separator tube functions.

____

____

52. Describe the function of the tourniquet. Include the appropriate distance from the puncture site a tourniquet should be placed and the recommended time it should be on the arm.

____

____

53. Discuss the criteria for determining whether a tourniquet is on correctly.

____

____

54. List the assets and limitations of the topical anesthetic EMLA.

____

____

55. Why should the tourniquet be released before removing the needle?

____

____

56. Why does the needle need to be held steady during the venipuncture procedure?

____

____

57. Name the three methods that can be used to obtain blood from a vein.

58. What are the most frequently used needle gauges for the Vacutainer system?

59. List the advantages of using the Vacutainer method.

60. Explain when a butterfly and syringe method would be used.

61. Describe the safety steps of discarding the needle after removing it from the arm with the Vacutainer method.

62. List three conditions that could cause a hematoma.

63. Describe the recommended procedure for transferring blood from a syringe into vacuum tubes.

64. Describe the procedure for determining the appropriate vein for venipuncture.

65. Identify and describe the function of each part of the syringe system.

66. Label the parts of the syringe.

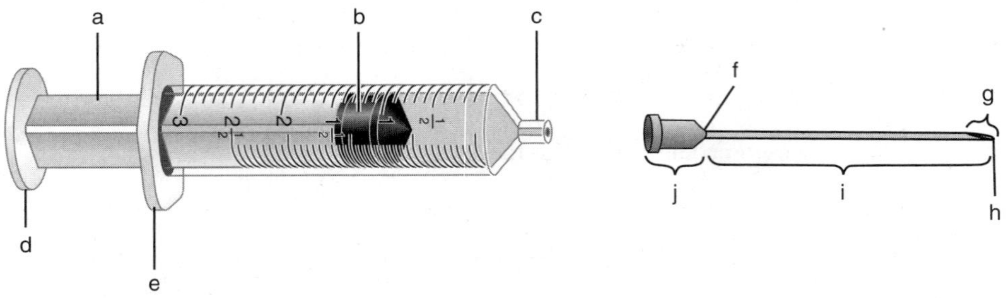

67. Identify and describe the function of each of the components of the butterfly system, including use of the Luer Adapter/Vacutainer method and the syringe method.

____

____

68. Label the supplies needed for the butterfly system.

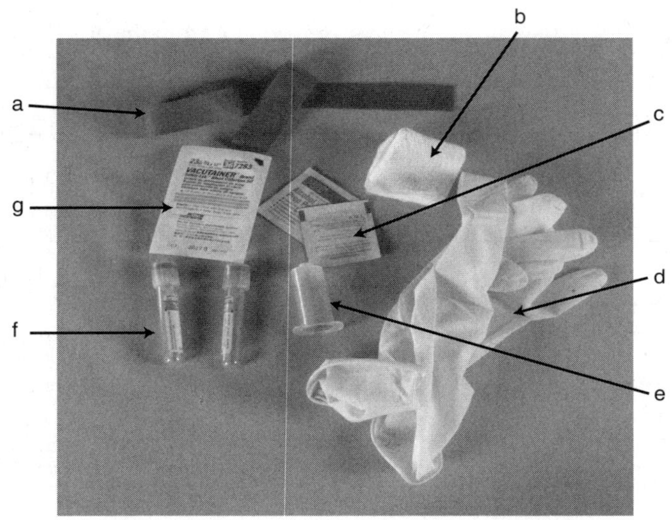

69. Identify two quality assurance steps related to vacuum tube selection.

____

____

70. Discuss the Needle Stick Safety and Prevention Act passed by Congress, which directed the Occupational Safety and Health Administration (OSHA) to revise the bloodborne pathogens standards to require employers to identify and use safer medical devices.

____

____

71. In the following case study steps, write **C** if the technique is correct or **I** if the technique is incorrect, and explain why in the space provided.
A medical assistant is performing a Vacutainer blood collection method.

_______ 1. The patient is told to sit on the end of the examination table.

____

_______ 2. The medical assistant washes his or her hands, puts on gloves, and then pops the top off of the index finger of the glove.

____

_______ 3. The tourniquet is applied, and the median cubital vein is determined for use; the tourniquet is then removed.

____

_______ 4. The chosen site is cleaned with 70% alcohol, working in concentric circles from the inside out, making sure to not backtrack. The tourniquet is then reapplied.

____

_______ 5. The nondominant hand anchors the vein.

____

_______ 6. The angle of the needle is 45 degrees as it enters the vein.

____

_______ 7. After the needle is removed, the safety device is immediately activated.

____

_______ 8. The needle is unscrewed from the holder and discarded in a sharps container, reusing the holder.

____

72. In the following scenario about the venipuncture method, circle the incorrect techniques. In the space provided, explain the repercussions that could occur from using the incorrect method.
A medical assistant examines an arm to determine the correct vein to use to obtain blood. The arm has very small veins. The medical assistant decides to use the Vacutainer method. The patient's name is determined by asking, "Are you Mrs. Jones?" The patient is then told to sit in a chair with an arm. All the tubes that will be drawn on this patient are prelabeled before the draw. After putting on the tourniquet approximately 3 inches above the puncture site, the arm is cleaned with 70% isopropyl alcohol, starting at the puncture site and moving in a concentric circle outward. The site is retouched by the phlebotomist without cleaning the finger. The needle is inserted into the vein at a 15-degree angle. The lavender tube is filled first, followed by the red tube and gray tube; the green tube is filled last. After the last tube is filled, the needle is removed from the vein, and the tourniquet is removed. Tubes are mixed approximately three times and placed in an upright position in the tray to be quickly taken to the lab to perform analytical testing.

____

____

____

____

____

____

____

73. Label all the venipuncture supplies in the figure below (see Figure 4-22 in the textbook).

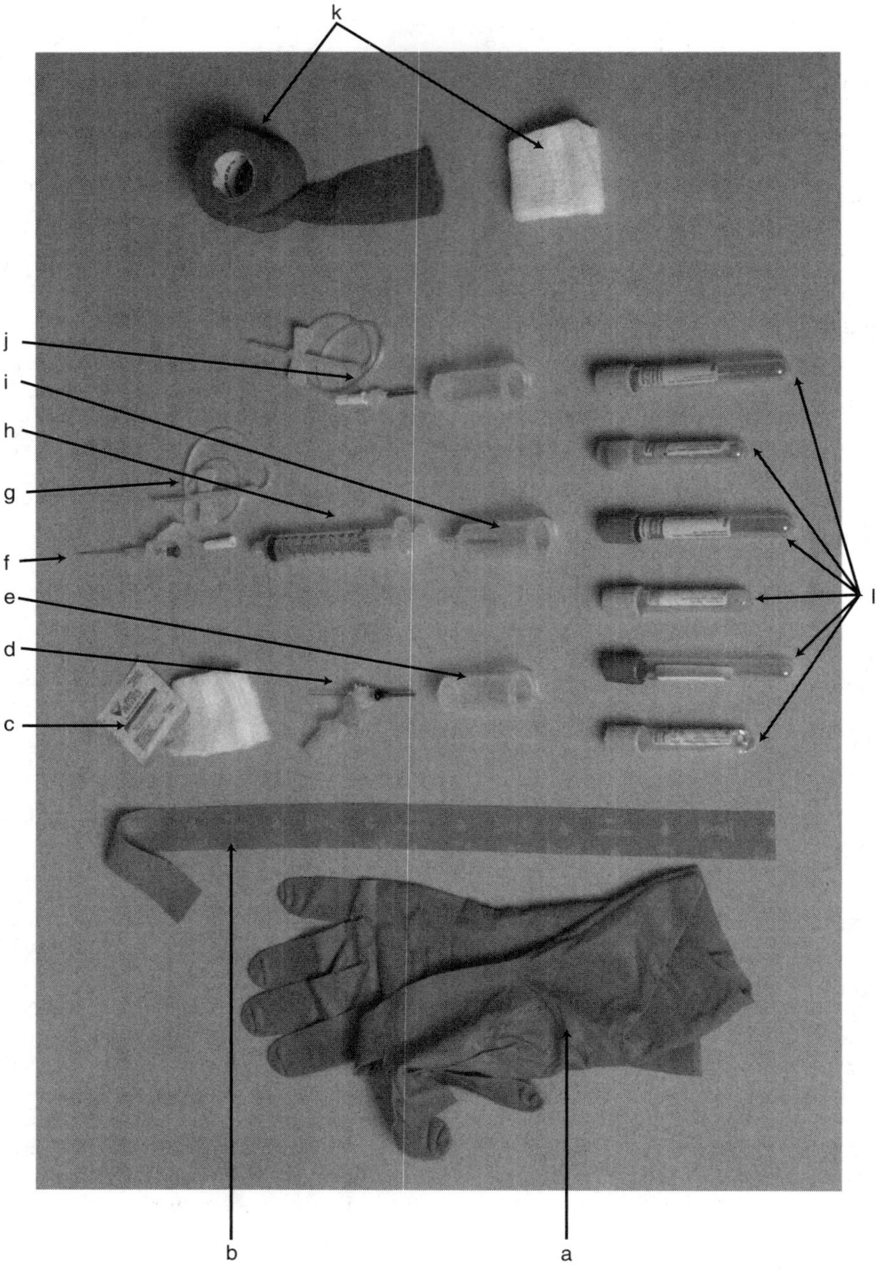

74. Internet activity: Visit one of the following Web sites, and present your findings to the class.
www.mchb.hrsa.gov (Maternal and Child Health Bureau of the Health Resources and Services Administration)
www.aap.org (American Academy of Pediatrics)
www.bd.com (Becton Dickinson)
www.nccls.org (National Committee for Clinical Laboratory Standards)
www.osha.gov (Occupational Safety and Health Administration)

ADVANCED CONCEPTS

75. The medical assistant is performing a Vacutainer procedure. The needle is inserted into the vein, and the vacuum tube is pushed into the Vacutainer holder. No blood is obtained. Discuss the possible reasons why this occurred.

____

____

____

76. During a venipuncture procedure, the patient becomes pale, sweats, and hyperventilates. Discuss what occurred and what should be done.

____

____

____

77. The plasma in the vacuum tube appears pink. Explain what this is, list three things that can cause it, and name three tests that can be affected by this condition.

____

____

____

78. After a needle was inserted into a patient's vein, the patient experienced a tingling sensation radiating down the arm. What occurred, and what should the phlebotomist do?

____

____

____

Procedure 4-1: Capillary Puncture Procedure

Person evaluated ______________________ Date ______________

Evaluated by ______________________ Score ______________

Outcome goal	To perform a capillary skin puncture with a retractable, nonreusable lancet
Conditions	Given the following supplies: - Sterile, disposable, retractable, nonreusable lancets (various lengths for the appropriate depth) - Microcollection containers, plastic capillary tubes (with anticoagulant) and sealers - Sterile gauze and 70% isopropyl alcohol pads in sterile packages - Gloves (latex and nonlatex for patients who are allergic) - Biohazard puncture-resistant sharps container - Warming devices, marking pen - Appropriate microcollection containers and/or testing devices depending on what test is ordered
Standards	Required time: 10 minutes Performance time ____________ Total possible points = ____________ Points earned = ____________
Evaluation Rubric Codes: **S** = Satisfactory, meets standard **U** = Unsatisfactory, fails to meet standard	
NOTE: Steps marked with an asterisk (*) are critical to achieve required competency.	

Preparation	Scores S	Scores U
*1. Identified patient and placed in proper position.		
- Had patient state name.		
- Confirmed identification with patient (birth date or picture ID).		
- Compared with requisition.		
2. Sanitized hands and put on gloves.		
3. Determined the most suitable puncture site and warmed the site.		
- A finger stick: third and fourth finger should be used, making the puncture on the lateral part of the fingertip (slightly to the side of center) and perpendicular to the fingerprint.		
- Newborn or infant (not walking): the medial or lateral plantar section of the foot should be used.		
- Warmed area by massaging the areas five or six times or applied a warmed towel, preemie diaper, or a commercially available device to the site for 3 to 5 minutes.		
Procedure	**S**	**U**
*4. Disinfected area over chosen site and assembled equipment.		
- Cleaned the site with 70% alcohol.		
- Allowed to dry without fanning or blowing on cleansed site.		

	S	U
- Assembled the capillary equipment needed, determining the appropriate lancet device to use according to the age and amount of blood needed.		
- Placed all supplies in close proximity to hand.		
5. Pressing hard, made a puncture in the cleaned area at the appropriate site.		
*6. Wiped away the first drop of blood.		
*7. Collected the blood in the proper container by the correct technique.		
- Collected free-flowing drops of blood; did not scoop, scrape, or squeeze the site.		
- If blood was collected in a capillary tube, held the tube horizontal to the site and did not have any air bubbles.		
Follow-up	**Scores**	
	S	**U**
8. Asked the patient to apply pressure to site for 3 to 5 minutes.		
9. Gently mixed microcontainers by tilting 8 to 10 times and labeled all tubes properly.		
- Marked date and time of draw, patient name, and initials or name of phlebotomist.		
- Placed capillary tubes in a vacuum tube and labeled the vacuum tube.		
*10. Checked site for bleeding and applied pressure bandage to site.		
- If bleeding continued after 5 minutes, contacted physician.		
- Checked if patient was allergic to bandages before application.		
- Informed parent, if patient is a child, to remove the adhesive bandage after bleeding is stopped because children may choke on it if swallowed.		
11. Determined whether patient was feeling well before dismissing.		
*12. Completed proper documentation on patient chart (see below).		
*13. Properly performed disposal and disinfection.		
- Disposed all sharps into biohazard sharps containers.		
- Disposed regulated medical waste into biohazard bags (gloves, gauze).		
- Disinfected test area and instruments according to OSHA guidelines.		
14. Sanitized hands.		
Total Points per Column		

Patient Name: ________________

Patient Chart Entry: (Include when, what, how, why, any additional information, and the signature of the person charting.)

____

____

____

Procedure 4-2: Heel Stick for Neonatal Screening Test Procedure

Person evaluated ______________________ Date ______________

Evaluated by ______________________ Score ______________

Outcome goal	Perform a capillary skin puncture with a retractable, nonreusable lancet
Conditions	Given the following supplies: - Gloves (preferably nonlatex for latex-sensitive patients) - Sterile gauze - Warming device - 70% isopropyl alcohol pads in sterile packages - Sterile, disposable, retractable, nonreusable neonatal lancets with no more than 2-mm depth - Neonatal screening filter paper
Standards	Required time: 15 minutes Performance time ________ Total possible points = ________ Points earned = ________
Evaluation Rubric Codes: **S** = Satisfactory, meets standard **U** = Unsatisfactory, fails to meet standard	
NOTE: Steps marked with an asterisk (*) are critical to achieve required competency.	

Preparation	**Scores** S	U
*1. Wash the hands if they are visibly soiled. If not, use an alcohol-based rub for routine decontamination. Apply the hand rub to the palm of one hand, and rub the hands together, covering all surfaces until dry.		
2. Correctly identify the newborn by using the three-way match, and fill out all the information required on the card.		
3. Applied gloves.		
4. Choose the appropriate site for the heel stick according to the guidelines.		
- Newborn or infant (not walking): the medial or lateral plantar section of the foot should be used.		
- Applied a warmed towel, preemie diaper, or a commercially available device to the site for 3 to 5 minutes.		
Procedure	**Scores** S	U
5. Clean the site with 70% isopropyl alcohol. Allow the alcohol to dry, and do not fan or blow on the site.		
6. With a gloved hand, place the lancet against the medial or lateral plantar surface of the heel of the foot.		
7. Place the blade slot area securely against the heel, and firmly and completely depress the lancet trigger.		
8. Gently wipe away the first drop of blood with sterile gauze or cotton ball.		
9. Apply gentle pressure with the thumb and ease intermittently as drops of blood form. Be sure to apply pressure in such a way that the incision site remains open.		

*10. The filter paper should be touched gently against the large blood drop, and in one step, a sufficient quantity of blood should soak through to completely fill a preprinted circle on the filter paper.		
- Do not reapply additional drops in the same circle.		
- The paper should not be pressed or smeared against the puncture site of the heel.		
- Blood should be applied only to one side of the filter paper, but both sides of the filter paper should be examined to ensure that the blood uniformly saturated the paper.		
11. After all five circles of blood have been collected from the heel of the newborn, the foot should be elevated above the body.		
NOTE: A minimum of three successful circles is needed by the laboratory to test for multiple metabolic disorders.		
12. A sterile gauze pad or cotton swab should be pressed against the puncture site until the bleeding stops.		
- It is not advisable to apply adhesive bandages over skin puncture sites on newborns.		

Follow-up	**Scores**	
	S	**U**
*13. Log and chart the procedure.		
14. Allow filter paper to dry thoroughly on a horizontal, level, nonabsorbent open surface for 3 hours at ambient temperature and away from direct sunlight.		
- Do not touch or smear blood on the filter paper, and do not contaminate the specimen card with cleaning chemicals or other substances.		
- Mail the thoroughly dried card (Fig. F in textbook) in the envelope provided by the health department.		
- Placed capillary tubes in a vacuum tube and labeled the vacuum tube.		
*15. Properly performed disposal and disinfection.		
- Disposed all sharps into biohazard sharps containers.		
- Disposed regulated medical waste into biohazard bags (gloves, gauze).		
- Disinfected test area and instruments according to OSHA guidelines.		
16. Sanitized hands.		
Total Points per Column		

Patient Name: ________________

Patient Chart Entry: (Include when, what, how, why, any additional information, and the signature of the person charting.)

____

____

____

Procedure 4-3: Vacutainer Method

Person evaluated ______________________ Date ______________

Evaluated by ______________________ Score ______________

Outcome goal	Perform a venipuncture by the Vacutainer method
Conditions	Given the following supplies: - Disposable gloves - Tourniquet - 70% isopropyl alcohol and sterile gauze pads - Vacutainer double-pointed needle and Vacutainer holder - Correct vacuum tubes for requested tests - Adhesive bandages - Test tube rack - Biohazard sharps containers and bags
Standards	Required time: 10 minutes Performance time ________ Total possible points = ________ Points earned = ________
Evaluation Rubric Codes: **S** = Satisfactory, meets standard **U** = Unsatisfactory, fails to meet standard	
NOTE: Steps marked with an asterisk (*) are critical to achieve required competency.	

Preparation	**Scores S**	**U**
*1. Identified and placed patient in proper position.		
- Had patient state name.		
- Confirmed identification with patient (birth date or picture ID).		
- Compared identification with requisition.		
2. Sanitized hands and put on gloves.		
3. Applied tourniquet and determined the most suitable puncture site.		
- Used sufficient pressure to stop venous flow but not arterial flow.		
- Palpated and determined size, depth, and direction of vein.		
4. Removed tourniquet, disinfected area over chosen site, and assembled equipment.		
- Cleansed the site with 70% alcohol in concentric circles from inside out.		
- Allowed to dry without fanning or blowing on cleansed site.		
- Connected the venipuncture assembly in a sterile manner.		
- Placed all supplies in close proximity to arm.		

Procedure	Scores S	Scores U
5. Reapplied tourniquet and instructed patient to make a fist (no pumping).		
*6. Disinfected gloved fingers if necessary to palpate site again.		
*7. Uncovered needle, anchored vein, and inserted needle.		
- Pulled skin taut with nondominant thumb 1 to 2 inches below and to the side of the puncture site.		
- Inserted needle ¼ to ½ inches distal to the vein with bevel up in one swift, continuous motion with dominant hand.		
*8. Pushed tube into needle holder.		
- Used the index and middle fingers of nondominant hand on both sides of the flange and pushed the tube with the thumb of the same hand.		
*9. Followed proper order of draw when filling, removing, and mixing the tubes.		
- Used thumb of nondominant hand against flange and pulled tube out with the fingers of the same hand.		
- Inverted each tube gently to mix blood with additives.		
- Removed the last tube to prevent blood dripping from needle.		
- Instructed patient to release fist.		
*10. Removed tourniquet before taking needle out of arm.		
*11. Placed sterile gauze over needle as it was pulled out and then applied pressure to site.		
- Did not press on the gauze until *after* the needle was removed.		
*12. Immediately activated needle safety device and discarded Vacutainer and needle as a unit into the sharps container.		

Follow-up	Scores S	Scores U
13. Asked the patient to apply pressure to site for 3 to 5 minutes.		
14. Gently mixed tubes by tilting 8 to 10 times and labeled all tubes properly.		
- Marked patient name, date and time of draw, and initials or name of phlebotomist.		
*15. Checked site for bleeding and applied pressure bandage to site.		
- If bleeding continued after 5 minutes, contacted physician.		
- Checked if patient was allergic to bandages before application.		
16. Determined if patient was feeling well before dismissing.		
17. Completed proper documentation on patient chart (see following page).		

*18. Properly disposed and disinfected materials.		
- Disposed all sharps into biohazard sharp containers.		
- Disposed regulated medical waste (e.g., gloves, gauze) into biohazard bags.		
- Disinfected test area and instruments according to OSHA guidelines.		
19. Sanitized hands.		
Total Points per Column		

Patient Name: ________________

Patient Chart Entry: (Include when, what, how, why, any additional information, and the signature of the person charting.)

____

____

____

Procedure 4-4: Syringe Method

Person evaluated ______________________ Date ______________

Evaluated by ______________________ Score______________

Outcome goal	Perform a venipuncture by the syringe method
Conditions	Given the following supplies: - Disposable gloves - Tourniquet - 70% isopropyl alcohol and sterile gauze pads - Proper-sized syringe and needle - Safety transfer device - Correct vacuum tubes for requested tests - Adhesive bandages - Test tube rack - Biohazard sharps containers and bags
Standards	Required time: 10 minutes Performance time ____________ Total possible points = ____________ Points earned = ____________
Evaluation Rubric Codes: **S** = Satisfactory, meets standard **U** = Unsatisfactory, fails to meet standard	
NOTE: Steps marked with an asterisk (*) are critical to achieve required competency.	

Preparation	Scores S	Scores U
*1. Identified and placed patient in proper position.		
- Had patient state name.		
- Confirmed identification with patient (birth date or picture ID).		
- Compared identification with requisition.		
2. Sanitized hands and put on gloves.		
3. Applied tourniquet and determined the most suitable puncture site.		
- Applied sufficient pressure to stop venous flow but not arterial flow.		
- Palpated and determined size, depth, and direction of vein.		
4. Removed tourniquet, disinfected area over chosen site, and assembled equipment.		
- Cleaned the site with 70% alcohol in concentric circles from inside out.		
- Allowed to dry without fanning or blowing on cleansed site.		
- Connected the syringe assembly in a sterile manner.		
- Placed all supplies in close proximity to arm.		
Procedure	**Scores S**	**Scores U**
*5. Reapplied tourniquet and instructed patient to make a fist (no pumping).		
- Disinfected gloved fingers if necessary to palpate site again.		

	S	U
*6. Removed needle cover, anchored vein, and inserted needle.		
- Pulled skin taut with nondominant thumb 1 to 2 inches distal to the site of the puncture.		
- Inserted needle ¼ to ½ inches distal to the vein with bevel up in one swift, continuous motion with dominant hand at the appropriate angle.		
*7. Gently pulled syringe plunger back.		
- Was careful to not pull out of the vein.		
- Instructed patient to release fist.		
*8. Removed tourniquet before taking needle out of arm.		
*9. Placed sterile gauze over needle as it was pulled out, then applied pressure to site.		
- Did not press on the gauze until after the needle was removed.		
*10. Immediately activated syringe needle safety device, unscrewed the needle, and discarded it into the sharps container.		
Follow-up	**Scores**	
	S	**U**
11. Asked the patient to apply pressure with gauze to site for 3 to 5 minutes.		
12. Filled the vacuum tubes in the proper order of draw by using a transfer safety device.		
- Did not push on the plunger.		
13. Gently mixed tubes by tilting 8 to 10 times and labeled all tubes properly.		
- Marked patient name, date and time of draw, and initials or name of phlebotomist.		
*14. Checked site for bleeding and applied pressure bandage to site.		
- If bleeding continued after 5 minutes, contacted physician.		
- Checked if patient was allergic to bandages before application.		
15. Determined if patient was feeling well before dismissing.		
16. Completed proper documentation on patient chart (see below).		
*17. Properly disposed and disinfected materials.		
- Disposed all sharps, including the transfer device/syringe, into biohazard sharps container.		
- Disposed regulated medical waste into biohazard bags (gloves, gauze).		
- Disinfected test area and instruments according to OSHA guidelines.		
18. Sanitized hands.		
Total Points per Column		

Patient Name ________________

Patient Chart Entry: (Include when, what, how, why, any additional information, and the signature of the person charting.)

____

____

____

Procedure 4-5: Two Butterfly Methods from a Hand and Training Model

Person evaluated ______________________ Date ______________

Evaluated by ______________________ Score ______________

Outcome goal	Perform a venipuncture by the butterfly method
Conditions	Given the following supplies: - Disposable gloves, tourniquet, 70% isopropyl alcohol and gauze pads - Winged butterfly set (Safety-Lock and/or Push Button) with syringe adapter and Vacutainer adapter - Proper-sized syringe or Vacutainer holder - Correct vacuum tubes for requested tests - Adhesive bandages - Test tube rack and biohazard sharps containers and bags
Standards	Required time: 10 minutes Performance time ______ Total possible points = ______ Points earned = ______
Evaluation Rubric Codes: **S** = Satisfactory, meets standard **U** = Unsatisfactory, fails to meet standard	
NOTE: Steps marked with an asterisk (*) are critical to achieve required competency.	

Preparation	**Scores**	
	S	**U**
*1. Identified and placed patient in proper position.		
- Had patient state name.		
- Confirmed identification with patient (birth date or picture ID).		
- Compared identification with requisition.		
2. Sanitized hands and put on gloves.		
3. Applied tourniquet and determined the most suitable puncture site.		
- Applied sufficient pressure to stop venous flow but not arterial flow.		
- Palpated and determined size, depth, and direction of vein.		
4. Removed tourniquet, disinfected area over chosen site, and assembled equipment.		
- Cleaned the site with 70% alcohol in concentric circles from inside out.		
- Allowed to dry without fanning or blowing on cleansed site.		
- Straightened out the butterfly tubing.		
- Connected the venipuncture butterfly assembly in a sterile manner to a syringe or a Vacutainer holder.		
- Pushed the plunger back and forth to break the seal if attaching a syringe.		
- Placed all supplies in close proximity to arm or hand.		

Procedure	Scores S	Scores U
*5. Reapplied the tourniquet and disinfected gloved fingers if necessary to palpate site again.		
*6. Removed needle sheath, anchored vein, and inserted needle.		
- Pulled skin taut with nondominant thumb 1 to 2 inches below and to the side of the puncture site.		
- Held the butterfly wings together with the dominant hand and inserted needle ¼ to ½ inches distal to the vein with bevel up in one swift, continuous motion with dominant hand at the appropriate angle.		
*7. Used the correct technique to obtain blood.		
- Gently pulled syringe plunger back if using syringe method.		
- Used the index and middle fingers of nondominant hand on both sides of the flange and pushed the tube into the holder with the thumb of the same hand if the Vacutainer method was used.		
*8. Tourniquet removed before taking needle out of arm.		
*9. Placed sterile gauze over needle as it was pulled out and then applied pressure to the site.		
- Did not press on the gauze until after the needle was removed.		
*10. Immediately activated butterfly needle safety device in a safe manner and disposed of butterfly apparatus properly (illustrations show how to activate the Safety Lock and the Push Button safety devices).		
- If Vacutainer method was used, the butterfly needle, tubing, and Vacutainer holder were placed in a biohazard sharps container.		
- If a syringe method was used, the syringe was removed from the butterfly tubing, and the butterfly needle and tubing were discarded into a biohazard sharps container.		

Follow-up	Scores S	Scores U
11. Asked the patient to apply pressure with gauze to site for 3 to 5 minutes.		
12. Filled the vacuum tubes in the proper order of draw by using a transfer safety device if syringe method was used.		
- Did not push on plunger; let vacuum fill the tube.		
13. Gently mixed tubes by tilting 8 to 10 times, and labeled all tubes properly.		
- Marked patient name, date and time of draw, and initials or name of phlebotomist.		
*14. Checked site for bleeding and applied pressure bandage to site.		
- If bleeding continued after 5 minutes, contacted physician.		
- Checked if patient was allergic to bandages before application.		
15. Determined if patient was feeling well before dismissing.		
16. Completed proper documentation on patient chart (see following page).		

*17. Properly disposed and disinfected equipment.		
- Disposed all sharps, including the transfer device and syringe (if syringe method was used), into biohazard sharps containers.		
- Disposed regulated medical waste (e.g., gloves, gauze) into biohazard bags.		
- Disinfected test area and instruments according to OSHA guidelines.		
18. Sanitized hands.		
Total Points per Column		

Patient Name: ________________

Patient Chart Entry: (Include when, what, how, why, any additional information, and the signature of the person charting.)

____

____

____

Vacuum Tube Exercise

Visualize the following picture:

- *Blue* sky is at the top and is the first tube to draw.
- The *red and gold* rays of the sun are on the horizon. They both must be drawn *after* the blue but *before* the remaining anticoagulant tubes.
- *Green* grassy hill is located below the sun rays.
- *Lavender* flowers are at the bottom of the hill growing above the rocks.
- *Gray* rocks are at the bottom of the picture because gray is the last tube to draw.

Next, fill in the blank boxes and missing words from Table 4-5 in the textbook. Cut the rows, mix them up, and then place back in order, or cut all the boxes and put them back together like a puzzle.

Colors of Picture and the Plastic Vacutainer Tubes Placed in Order of Draw from Top to Bottom		Additives	Laboratory Uses
blue ________	blue topped	________	________
red rays and gold ________	________ topped ________	clot activator in plastic tubes (red *glass* tubes do not have clot activator)	both yield serum commonly used for testing blood ________
	gold topped ________	________ and ________	
________ grass	green topped	________ (with lithium or sodium)	special tests such as ________
lavender flowers	lavender topped	________	________
gray ________	________	oxalate	for ________ testing

5 Hematology

VOCABULARY REVIEW

Match each hematology term with the correct definition.

A. anisocytosis
B. baso
C. differentiate
D. eosin
E. erythroblasts
F. formed elements
G. granulocytes
H. hematologists
I. hematopoiesis
J. hemocytoblast
K. macrophages
L. megakaryocyte
M. myeloblast
N. nongranulocytes
O. -phil
P. poikilocytosis
Q. polymorphonuclear
R. reticulocytes
S. thrombocytes

________ 1. Large nuclear cell in the bone marrow that fragments its cytoplasm to become platelets

________ 2. Stem cell that develops into the three kinds of granulocytes

________ 3. Abnormally shaped

________ 4. Acid

________ 5. Alkaline

________ 6. Also called rubriblasts, which become red blood cells

________ 7. Attraction

________ 8. Blood production

________ 9. Cells and cell fragments that can be viewed under the microscope

________ 10. Specialists who evaluate the cellular elements of blood microscopically and analytically

________ 11. Large, engulfing cells in the tissues that come from monocytes

________ 12. Lymphocyte and monocyte group

________ 13. Many-shaped nucleus; also called PMN or seg

________ 14. Neutrophils, basophils, and eosinophils group

________ 15. Newly released red blood cells in the blood that still contain some nuclear DNA

________ 16. Stem cell capable of becoming any of the blood cells

________ 17. To change and become something different

________ 18. Variances in red blood cell size

________ 19. Platelets

Match each coagulation or pathology term with the correct definition.

A. anemia
B. embolus
C. fibrinogen, prothrombin
D. hemolysis
E. hemostasis
F. hypoxemia
G. leukemia
H. leukocytosis
I. leukopenia
J. polycythemia
K. red blood cell indices
L. coagulation
M. rouleaux formation
N. thrombosis
O. vitamin K
P. differential count
Q. polychromia

_______ 20. A critical element in the production of prothrombin

_______ 21. A traveling clot

_______ 22. Abnormal condition of increased red blood cells

_______ 23. Abnormal decrease in white blood cells

_______ 24. Abnormal increase in white blood cells

_______ 25. Abnormal condition of clotting

_______ 26. Condition in which the red blood cell or hemoglobin levels are below normal

_______ 27. Destruction of the red blood cells

_______ 28. Lack of oxygen in the blood

_______ 29. Like stacked chips

_______ 30. Mathematic ratios of the three red blood cell tests (hemoglobin, hematocrit, and red blood cell count)

_______ 31. Blood's ability to maintain the balance of initiating a clotting response to stop bleeding and at the same time prevent the blood from forming an unwanted stationary clot

_______ 32. Two plasma proteins involved in clotting

_______ 33. Percentage of the five kinds of white blood cells

_______ 34. Cancer of the white blood cells

_______ 35. Increase in color (based on hemoglobin concentration)

_______ 36. Process of clotting

FUNDAMENTAL CONCEPTS

37. Blood collected from a _______________ or a _______________ may be used for routine hematologic procedures.

38. The anticoagulated Vacutainer tube containing _______________ with a _______________ top is used for most hematology tests.

39. Match each blood component with its associated characteristic.

_______ basophil
_______ erythrocyte
_______ monocyte
_______ neutrophil
_______ platelet
_______ lymphocyte
_______ eosinophil

A. Able to engulf foreign matter, especially bacteria
B. Increases in number during allergic reactions
C. Can differentiate into a T cell or B cell
D. Enters the tissues to mediate the inflammatory response
E. Gathers around the site of a damaged blood vessel and releases chemicals to stimulate clot formation
F. Carries oxygen from the lungs to the cells of the body
G. Becomes a macrophage when it leaves the blood to clean up debris in the tissues

40. Label the missing elements of the following hematopoiesis chart (see Figure 5-3 in the textbook).

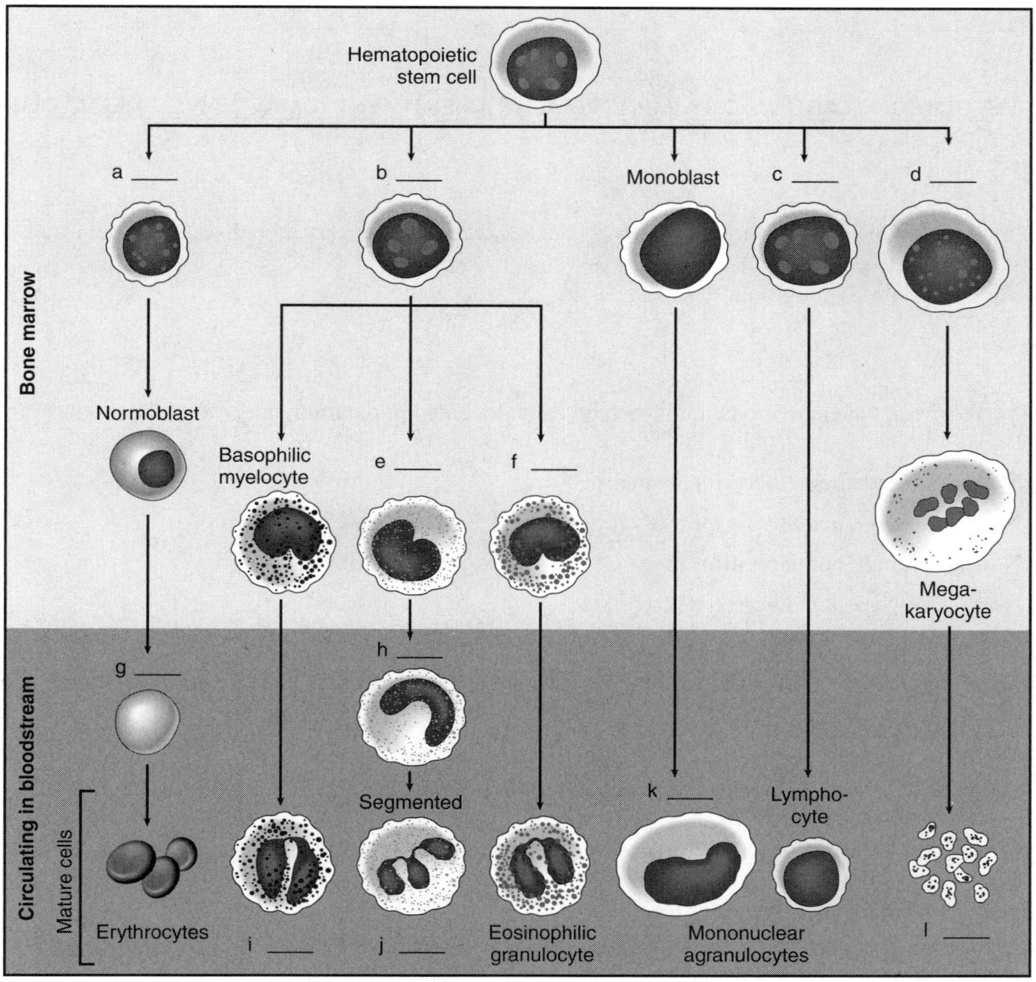

Preparation of a Blood Smear

41. A properly done blood smear will have a ________________ edge at the thin end of the slide and a section containing well-distributed blood cells in the ________________ of the slide.

42. Blood smears are observed under the ________________ lens.

43. When identifying cells, what three characteristics should the technician observe? (Hint: *The RBC Atlas* and *WBC Atlas* describe the general characteristics to observe in blood cells.)

____

____

Hemostasis

44. Explain the involvement of each of the following as they pertain to hemostasis.

Blood vessels ________________________________

Platelets ________________________________

Clotting factors ________________________________

Anticoagulants ________________________________

45. What is the difference between a thrombus and an embolus? ______________________________

____

PROCEDURES: CLINICAL LABORATORY IMPROVEMENT AMENDMENT (CLIA)–WAIVED HEMATOLOGY TESTS

Hemoglobin

46. The two main components of hemoglobin are ______________________ and ______________________.

47. What is the function of hemoglobin? ______________________________

Hematocrit

48. Match the following average hematocrit percentages to each population, and note the highest to the lowest averages.

_____ Normal average hematocrit for women	a. 56%
_____ Normal average hematocrit for a 6-year-old child	b. 42%
_____ Normal average hematocrit for men	c. 38%
_____ Normal average hematocrit for newborns	d. 47%

49. If a sample of capillary blood is used for the microhematocrit, the capillary tube must contain a(n)

______________________.

50. One condition in which a low hematocrit value may be found is ______________________________.

51. True or false: Spun hematocrits should be performed in duplicate. ______________________________

52. Label the layers of the spun hematocrit tube.

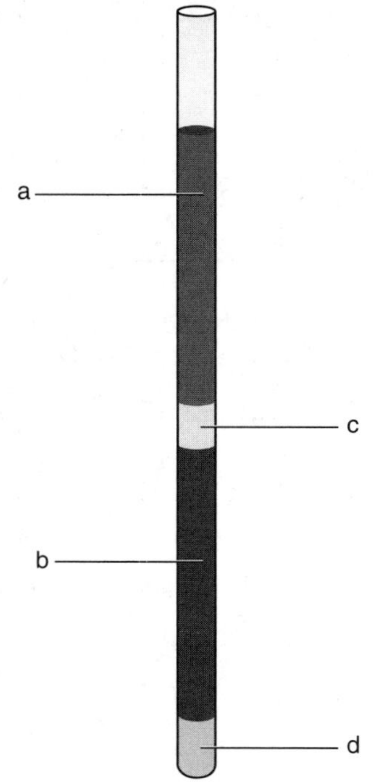

Erythrocyte Sedimentation Rate

53. What medical conditions can cause an increased erythrocyte sedimentation rate?

54. What technical interferences would cause an increased erythrocyte sedimentation rate?

Prothrombin Time

55. Describe the role of prothrombin in blood coagulation.

56. Explain the major use of the prothrombin time test.

57. Match each test with its reference range.

_______ hemoglobin	a. 36% to 55%
_______ hematocrit	b. 0 to 20 mm/hr
_______ ProTime	c. 12 to 18 g/dL
_______ ESR	d. approx. 9 to 18 seconds, or 2 to 2.5 INR

58. Label the Hemocue equipment and supplies (see Procedure 5-2 in the textbook).

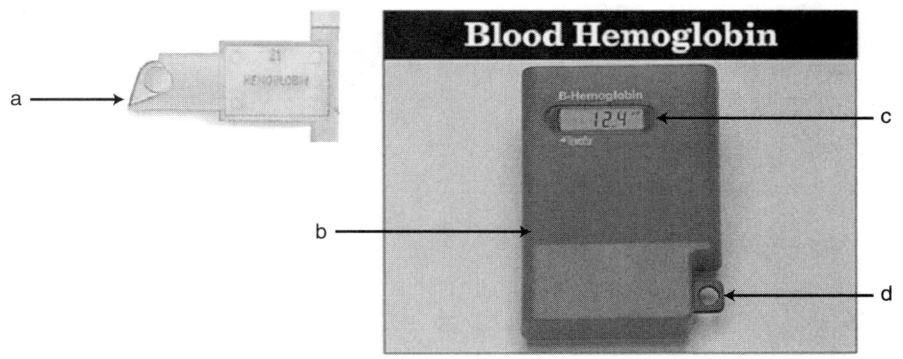

After approximately 15–45 seconds the result is displayed.

59. Label the SEDIPLAST ESR supplies (see Procedure 5-5 in the textbook).

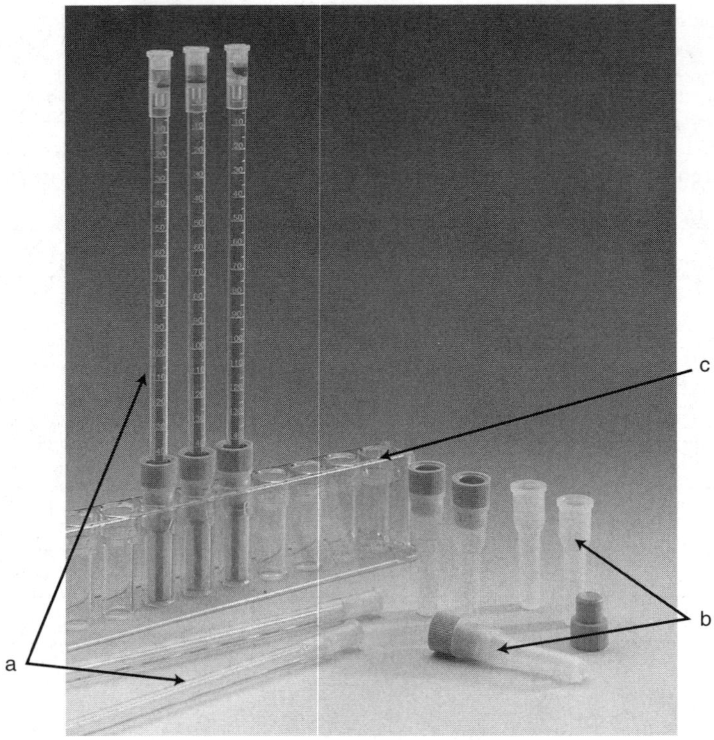

ADVANCED CONCEPTS: COMPLETE BLOOD COUNT

60. List the seven tests involved in the complete blood count.

____

____

____

____

____

____

____

61. What changes in blood cell size are caused by deficiency of vitamin B_{12}? (Hint: Look under "Anemias" in the textbook.)

____

____

62. List two conditions in which anisocytosis is found. (Hint: Look under "Anemias" in the textbook.)

____

____

63. Match the red blood cell indexes to their reference ranges. (Hint: See Table 5-3 or 5-4, and note the units associated with each test.)

_______ MCV   a. 26 to 34 pg

_______ MCH   b. 31% to 37% or g/dL

_______ MCHC   c. 82 to 98 μm^3 or fL

64. Hypochromic, microcytic red blood cells have a (higher or lower) ______________________ MCV and (higher or lower) ______________________ MCHC.

65. Why does anemia or thrombocytopenia develop in patients with leukemia? (Hint: Consider where and how hematopoiesis occurs.)

____

____

66. Name one cause of eosinophilia. (Review granulocyte functions in "Fundamental Concepts.")

____

____

67. Name one cause of neutrophilia. (Review granulocyte functions in "Fundamental Concepts.")

____

____

70. Match the cell with its differential reference percentage according to Table 5-3 in your textbook, and note the highest to the lowest.

_______ band   a. 3% to 9%

_______ lymphocyte   b. 50% to 65%

_______ neutrophil   c. 0% to 7%

_______ monocyte   d. 0% to 1%

_______ eosinophil   e. 25% to 40%

_______ basophil   f. 1% to 3%

Procedure 5-1: Diff Staining Procedure

Person evaluated ______________________ Date ______________

Evaluated by ______________________ Score ______________

Outcome goal	Demonstrate the proper staining of a blood smear
Conditions	Given the following supplies: - Quick Diff stain: fixative, red eosin dye, blue baso dye; - staining rack; - water source (bottled or running water); - bibulous paper - Personal protective equipment – gown & gloves
Standards	Required time: 10 minutes Performance time ________ Total possible points = ________ Points earned = ________
Evaluation Rubric Codes: **S** = Satisfactory, meets standard **U** = Unsatisfactory, fails to meet standard	

Preparation	**Scores S**	**Scores U**
1. Put on personal protective equipment (PPE).		
Procedure	**S**	**U**
2. Dip the slide in fixative three to five times and allow it to dry completely.		
3. Dip the slide into the red eosin dye three to five times.		
4. Let the excess dye run off and blot the rest away with absorbent paper.		
5. Dip the slide into the blue baso dye three to five times.		
6. After the blue dye is blotted away, rinse the slide thoroughly with water on both sides and allow it to air dry. It may also be pressed between two bibulous papers to help remove the water.		
Follow-up	**S**	**U**
*7. Observe the slide under the oil immersion lens of the microscope. The challenge is to find the WBCs.		
- Refer to the microscope skill sheet 2-1 in Chapter 2 for the proper steps to bring the slide into focus under the oil immersion lens.		
- The cells and platelets will be enlarged 1000 times (100× oil objective times the 10× ocular lens).		
- The slide will show predominantly RBCs with some small platelet clumps throughout.		
- The two most commonly found WBCs are segmented neutrophils and small lymphocytes.		
- See Table 5-1 for assistance in identifying the WBCs.		
Total Points per Column		

Procedure 5-2: Hemoglobin: HemoCue Method

Person evaluated ______________________________ Date ____________________

Evaluated by ______________________________ Score ____________________

Outcome goal	To perform FDA-approved hemoglobin waived test following the most current OSHA safety guidelines and applying the correct quality control
Conditions	Given - Control cuvette - Microcuvette testing devices - Liquid controls: high and low - Alcohol, gauze, safety lancets, and bandage
Standards	Required time = 10 minutes Performance time = ____________ Total possible points = ____________ Points earned = ____________
Evaluation Rubric Codes: **S** = Satisfactory, meets standard **U** = Unsatisfactory, fails to meet standard	
NOTE: Steps marked with an asterisk (*) are critical to achieve required competency.	

Preparation: Preanalytical Phase	Scores S	Scores U
A. Test information		
- Kit or instrument method: **HemoCue hemoglobin**		
- Manufacturer: **HemoCue**		
- Proper storage (e.g., temperature, light): **cuvettes stored at room temperature**		
- Lot number on cuvette container: ____________		
- Expiration date: ____________ **opened container is stable for 3 months**		
- Test flow chart: ________ yes ________ no		
B. Specimen information		
- Type of specimen: **capillary blood or EDTA tube blood**		
- Testing device: **microcuvette test device**		
C. Personal protective equipment: **gloves, gown, sharps, and biohazard**		
D. Assembled all the above, sanitized hands, and applied personal protective equipment.		
Procedure: Analytical Phase	**Scores S**	**Scores U**
E. Performed/observed quality control		
1. Quantitative testing controls		
- Calibration check: **used control cuvette for optics check**		
- Control levels: high ____________ low ____________		

F. Performed patient test	S	U
1. Followed proper steps (from test flow chart).		
2. Properly obtained sufficient drop of blood.		
- Wiped away first drop and allowed new drop to form.		
3. Filled cuvette completely in one continuous process; did not top off.		
4. Wiped off excess blood on outside of cuvette immediately.		
- Avoided pulling out blood by contacting tip of cuvette.		
5. Visually inspected for air bubbles and loss of blood from cuvette.		
6. Placed filled cuvette into the cuvette holder and pushed holder into the measuring position.		
7. Result displayed after 30 to 60 seconds.		
***Accurate Results** ________ **Instructor Confirmation** ________		

Follow-up: Postanalytical Phase	Scores	
	S	U
*G. Proper documentation		
1. On control log: ________ yes ________ no		
2. On patient log: ________ yes ________ no		
3. Documented on patient chart (see below).		
4. Identified critical values and took appropriate steps to notify physician. - Hemoglobin expected values: Adult men = 13.0 to 18 g/dL Adult women = 11.0 to 16.0 g/dL Infants = 10.0 to 14.0 g/dL Children = increase to adult		
H. Proper disposal and disinfection		
1. Disposed all sharps into biohazard sharps containers.		
2. Disposed all other regulated medical waste into biohazard bags.		
3. Disinfected test area and instruments according to OSHA guidelines.		
4. Sanitized hands after removing gloves.		
Totals Counts per Column		

Patient name: ________________________

Patient Chart Entry: (Include when, what, why, any additional information, and the signature of the person charting.)

____

____

____

Procedure 5-3: Hematocrit: General Procedure

Person evaluated ______________________ Date ______________

Evaluated by ______________________ Score ______________

Outcome goal	Perform FDA-approved hematocrit waived test following the most current OSHA safety guidelines and applying the correct quality control
Conditions	Supplies required: - Plastic capillary pipettes with anticoagulant - Sealant clay (e.g., Critoseal) or self-sealing capillary pipettes - Liquid controls: high and low - Gloves, gown, alcohol, gauze, and lancets - Hematocrit centrifuge with built-in reader and/or variable reader
Standards	Required time = 15 minutes Performance time = ____________ Total possible points = ____________ Points earned = ____________
Evaluation Rubric Codes: **S** = Satisfactory, meets standard **U** = Unsatisfactory, fails to meet standard	
NOTE: Steps marked with an asterisk (*) are critical to achieve required competency.	

Preparation: Preanalytical Phase	**Scores S**	**U**
A. Test information		
- Manufacturer: **Adams Readocrit (or other)**		
- Proper storage of pipettes and sealant (e.g., temperature, light): **room temperature**		
- Expiration date: **(2 years or 30 days after opened)**		
- Package insert or test flow chart available: ________ yes ________ no		
B. Specimen information		
- Type of specimen: **capillary blood or venous blood in EDTA tube**		
- Specimen testing device: **two capillary tubes filled at least halfway**		
C. Personal protective equipment: **gloves, gown, face shield**		
D. Assembled all the above, sanitized hands, and applied personal protective equipment.		
Procedure: Analytical Phase	**Scores S**	**U**
E. Performed/observed quality control		
1. Quantitative testing controls		
- **HemataCHEK reference control**		
- Control levels: high ____________ low ____________ normal ____________		

F. Perform patient test	S	U
1. Collected two heparin anticoagulated capillary tubes with blood from a finger or an EDTA tube of blood.		
- Hold the capillary tube in a horizontal position or slightly tilted down to allow capillary action to pull the blood into the tube, as shown in Figure A.		
- Avoid allowing bubbles into your specimen, and fill exactly to the line if using a built-in centrifuge scale or at least ½ full if using a variable reader.		
2. Collected whole blood into capillary tubes and sealed one end by pressing and turning in sealant, tapped the sealed end, or held presealed tube in vertical position for 15 seconds.		
3. Placed the tubes opposite each other with their clay ends toward the outside of the hematocrit centrifuge to create a balanced centrifuge.		
4. Locked the cover firmly against the capillary tubes to prevent breaking, and centrifuged for 5 minutes.		
5. Used the built-in scale or the variable scales to adjust the total volume (starting where the clay meets the cells and where the plasma meets the air at the top); determined the percentage of the total volume occupied by the red cells based on where they aligned with the plasma on the scale that is being used.		
6. Checked both readings to see if they were within 2% of each other, and recorded the average of the two tubes.		
***Accurate Results** ____________ **Instructor Confirmation** ____________		

Follow-up: Postanalytical Phase	**Scores**	
	S	**U**
*G. Proper documentation		
1. On control log: ____________ yes ____________ no		
2. On patient log: ____________ yes ____________ no		
3. Documented on patient chart (see following page).		
4. Identified critical values and took appropriate steps to notify physician. - Hematocrit expected values: Adult men = 42% to 52% Adult women = 36% to 48% Infants = 32% to 38% Children = increase to adult levels		

H. Proper disposal and disinfection		
1. Disposed all sharps into biohazard sharps containers.		
2. Disposed all other regulated medical waste into biohazard bags.		
3. Disinfected test area and instruments according to OSHA guidelines.		
4. Sanitized hands after removing gloves.		
Totals Counts per Column		

Patient Name: ______________________________

Patient Chart Entry: (Include when, what, why, any additional information, and the signature of the person charting.)

____

____

Procedure 5-4: Hematocrit: HemataSTAT Method

Person evaluated ______________________________ Date ______________________

Evaluated by ______________________________ Score ______________________

Outcome goal	To perform FDA-approved hematocrit waived test following the most current OSHA safety guidelines and applying the correct quality control
Conditions	Supplies required: - Plastic capillary pipettes with anticoagulant - Sealant clay (i.e., Critoseal) - Liquid controls: high and low - Gloves, gown, alcohol, gauze, and lancets
Standards	Required time = 15 minutes Performance time = __________ Total possible points = __________ Points earned = __________
Evaluation Rubric Codes: **S** = Satisfactory, meets standard **U** = Unsatisfactory, fails to meet standard	
NOTE: Steps marked with an asterisk (*) are critical to achieve required competency.	

Preparation: Preanalytical Phase	**Scores**	
	S	**U**
A. Test information		
- Kit or instrument method: **HemataSTAT II**		
- Manufacturer: **Separation Technology, Inc. (STI)**		
- Proper storage (e.g., temperature, light): **room temperature**		
- Expiration date: **(2 years or 30 days after opened)**		
- Package insert or test flow chart available: ________ yes ________ no		
B. Specimen information		
- Type of specimen: **capillary blood or venous blood in EDTA tube**		
- Specimen testing device: **two capillary tubes filled at least halfway**		
C. Personal protective equipment: **gloves, gown, face shield**		
D. Assembled all the above, sanitized hands, and applied personal protective equipment.		
Procedure: Analytical Phase	**Scores**	
	S	**U**
E. Performed/observed quality control		
1. Quantitative testing controls		
- HemataCHEK reference control		
- Control levels: high __________ low __________ normal __________		

F. Perform patient test	S	U
1. Followed proper steps (from test flow chart).		
2. Collected whole blood into capillary tubes and sealed one end by pressing and turning in sealant, and then tapped the sealed end. Or, held self-sealant tube vertical for 15 seconds.		
3. Inserted the sealed end of capillary tube into the HemataSTAT rotor tube holder.		
4. Closed centrifuge lid, locked latch, and pressed "RUN" to spin for 60 seconds.		
5. Waited for beeps, then unlocked latch and opened lid.		
6. Moved slider and sealed end of capillary tube to far left side of reader tray and rotated tube so entire "RED CELL/PLASMA" diagonal interface could be seen.		
7. Pressed "ENT" to read tube.		
8. Moved the slider black line to "SEALANT/RED CELL" interface and pressed "ENT."		
9. Moved the slider black line to "RED CELL/PLASMA" interface and pressed "ENT."		
10. Moved slider black line to "PLASMA/AIR" interface, pressed "ENT," noted result.		
11. Repeated steps 6 to 10 with second tube.		
- Result must be within 2% agreement of first reading.		
- Recorded the average of the two readings.		
***Accurate Results** ____________ **Instructor Confirmation** ____________		

Follow-up: Postanalytical Phase	**Scores**	
	S	**U**
*G. Proper documentation		
1. On control log: ____________ yes ____________ no		
2. On patient log: ____________ yes ____________ no		
3. Documented on patient chart (see following page).		
4. Identified critical values and took appropriate steps to notify physician.		
- Hematocrit expected values: Adult men = 42% to 52% Adult women = 36% to 48% Infants = 32% to 38% Children = increase to adult levels		
H. Proper disposal and disinfection		
1. Disposed all sharps into biohazard sharps containers.		
2. Disposed all other regulated medical waste into biohazard bags.		
3. Disinfected test area and instruments according to OSHA guidelines.		
4. Sanitized hands after removing gloves.		
Totals Counts per Column		

Patient Name: ______________________________

Patient Chart Entry: (Include when, what, why, any additional information, and the signature of the person charting.)

____

____

Procedure 5-5: ESR: SEDIPLAST System Procedure

Person evaluated ______________________ Date ______________

Evaluated by ______________________ Score ______________

Outcome goal	To perform FDA-approved ESR waived test following the most current OSHA safety guidelines and applying the correct quality control
Conditions	Supplies needed: - Plastic Westergren pipette graduated from 0 to 200 mm - SEDIPLAST vials with citrate diluent - Westergren rack for holding the pipettes - Disposal transfer pipette - Timer - Gloves, gown, face shield
Standards	Required time = 70 minutes Performance time = ____________ Total possible points = ____________ Points earned = ____________
Evaluation Rubric Codes: **S** = Satisfactory, meets standard **U** = Unsatisfactory, fails to meet standard	
NOTE: Steps marked with an asterisk (*) are critical to achieve required competency.	

Preparation: Preanalytical Phase	Scores	
	S	**U**
A. Test information		
- Kit or instrument method: **SEDIPLAST**		
- Manufacturer: **Polymedco, Inc.**		
- Proper storage (e.g., temperature, light): **room temperature**		
- Lot number on package: ______________		
- Expiration date: ______________		
- Package insert or test flow chart available: ________ yes ________ no		
B. Personal protective equipment: **gloves, gown, face shield**		
C. Proper specimen used for test		
- Type of specimen: **fresh EDTA whole blood up to 2 hours or refrigerated blood up to 6 hours**		
- Specimen testing device: **SEDIPLAST vial and pipette**		
D. Assembled all the above, sanitized hands, and applied personal protective equipment.		
Procedure: Analytical Phase	**Scores**	
	S	**U**
E. Performed/observed quality control methods: not applicable.		
F. Performed patient test.		

1. Removed stopper on vial and filled the vial with blood to indicated mark with a disposable transfer pipette (0.8 mL of blood needed).		
2. Replaced vial stopper and inverted vial several times to mix.		
3. Placed vial in SEDIPLAST rack on a level surface free of vibrations and jarring.		
4. Pressed the disposable SEDIPLAST pipette gently through the stopper with a twisting motion and continued to press until the pipette rested on the bottom of the vial (the pipette auto-zeros the blood, and any excess flows into the closed reservoir compartment at the top of the pipette).		
5. Set the timer for 1 hour, and let specimen stand undisturbed.		
6. After 1 hour read the numeric results of the ESR (used the scale at the top of the pipette to measure the distance from the top of the plasma to the top of the red blood cells).		
***Accurate Results** ________ **Instructor Confirmation** ________		
Follow-up: Postanalytical Phase	**Scores**	
	S	**U**
*G. Proper documentation		
1. On patient log: ________ yes ________ no		
2. Documented on patient chart (see below).		
3. Identified critical values, and took appropriate steps to notify physician.		
- ESR expected values: Men < 50 years = 0 to 15 mm/hr Men > 50 years = 0 to 20 mm/hr Women < 50 years = 0 to 20 mm/hr Women > 50 years = 0 to 30 mm/hr		
H. Proper disposal and disinfection		
1. Disposed all sharps into biohazard sharps containers.		
2. Disposed all other regulated medical waste into biohazard bags.		
3. Disinfected test area and instruments according to OSHA guidelines.		
4. Sanitized hands after removing gloves.		
Totals Counts per Column		

Patient name: ________________

Patient Chart Entry: (Include when, what, why, any additional information, and the signature of the person charting.)

____

____

Procedure 5-6: Prothrombin Time INRatio (HemoSense) Method

Person evaluated ______________________________ Date ______________________

Evaluated by ______________________________ Score ______________________

Outcome goal	To perform FDA-approved prothrombin waived test following the most current OSHA safety guidelines and applying correct quality control
Conditions	Supplies needed: - Gloves - Lancet with 21 gauge - Alcohol, gauze, and bandage for capillary puncture site care - INRatio test strips (at room temperature and sealed in foil container until within 10 minutes of testing) - INRatio meter with digital readout screen that guides the operator through the procedure - Biohazard sharps container
Standards	Required time = 10 minutes Performance time = __________ Total possible points = __________ Points earned = __________
Evaluation Rubric Codes: **S** = Satisfactory, meets standard **U** = Unsatisfactory, fails to meet standard	
NOTE: Steps marked with an asterisk (*) are critical to achieve required competency.	

Preparation: Preanalytical Phase	**Scores S**	**Scores U**
A. Test information.		
- Kit or instrument method: **INRatio.**		
- Manufacturer: **HemoSense.**		
- Proper storage (e.g., temperature, light): **foil-pouched test strips are refrigerated and must come to room temperature before opening.**		
- Expiration date: ______________________		
- Lot number on strip: ______________________		
- Package insert or test flow chart available: __________ yes __________ no.		
B. Personal protective equipment: **gloves, gown, face shield.**		
C. Proper specimen used for test.		
- Type of specimen: **fingerstick blood from a finger that has been warmed and gently massaged.**		
D. Assembled all the above, sanitized hands, and applied personal protective equipment.		
Procedure: Analytical Phase	**Scores S**	**Scores U**
E. Performed/observed quality control.		
- Quantitative testing controls.		

- Calibration check: **INRatio instrument and strips are precalibrated; no additional calibration is required.**		
- Control levels: **Each test cuvette has three channels that run a level I control, a level II control, and the patient test simultaneously.**		
F. Performed patient test.		
1. Turned on the INRatio meter by pressing any button; meter was on a level service and was not moved during testing.		
2. After self-test, the meter read "INSERT STRIP."		
3. Opened a test strip foil pouch, and removed the test strip; inserted the strip into the meter with "INRatio" readable at the bottom of the test strip (Fig. B in textbook).		
4. Checked that the strip code matched the one on the test strip pouch when "STRIP CODE ####" appeared in the display.		
- If it did, pressed the OK key.		
- If it did not, pressed the UP/DOWN button to change the first digit; pressed OK to enter the new digit; repeated for each new digit until the instrument and the strip codes matched and then pressed OK to finalize the code.		
- Meter then read "WARMING UP."		
5. Prepared the finger by warming, disinfecting, and drying thoroughly.		
- *Waited for the beep* and the prompt "APPLY SAMPLE"; a green sample light will appear through the test strip sample well.		
6. Incised the finger with the lancet.		
- Wiped away the first drop.		
- Formed a large, hanging drop using gentle continuous pressure.		
7. Applied the hanging drop to the sample well (where the green light shines through the test strip).		
8. Waited while the meter performed the test and calculated the results; message "TESTING SAMPLE" displayed.		
9. The meter beeped, and the results appeared on the display when the test was complete.		
- If an error message occurred, referred to the INRatio User's Guide for proper action.		
10. Read and recorded the INR and PT seconds from the digital screen.		
***Accurate Results INR** ____________ **PT** ____________ **Instructor Confirmation** ____________		
Follow-up: Postanalytical Phase	**Scores**	
	S	**U**
*G. Proper documentation		
1. On patient log: ____________ yes ____________ no		
2. Documented on patient chart (see following page).		

3. Identified critical values and took appropriate steps to notify physician. ProTime expected values for normal and therapeutic whole blood:		

	INR	PT (in seconds)
Normal	0.8–1.2	6.5 to 11.9 seconds for INRatio
Low anticoagulation	1.5–2.0	varies with method used
Moderate anticoagulation	2.0–3.0	varies with method used
High anticoagulation	2.5–4.0	varies with method used

H. Proper disposal and disinfection		
1. Disposed all sharps into biohazard sharps containers.		
2. Disposed all other regulated medical waste into biohazard bags.		
3. Disinfected test area and instruments according to OSHA guidelines.		
4. Sanitized hands after removing gloves.		
Totals Counts per Column		

Patient Name: ______________________________

Patient Chart Entry: (Include when, what, why, any additional information, and the signature of the person charting.)

____

____

6 Chemistry

VOCABULARY REVIEW

Match each definition with the correct term.

_______ 1. endogenous cholesterol
_______ 2. glycogen
_______ 3. exogenous cholesterol
_______ 4. catalysts
_______ 5. hyperinsulinemia
_______ 6. glycosylated Hgb
_______ 7. hyperlipidemia
_______ 8. insulin
_______ 9. glucagon
_______ 10. trans fats
_______ 11. ions
_______ 12. glycosuria
_______ 13. atherosclerosis
_______ 14. panels
_______ 15. dyslipidemia
_______ 16. carbohydrates
_______ 17. definitive diagnosis
_______ 18. hyperglycemia
_______ 19. clinical diagnosis
_______ 20. ketoacidosis
_______ 21. noncarbohydrate energy sources

A. Chemicals that produce specific changes in other substances without being changed themselves
B. Groups of tests providing information on particular organs or body metabolism
C. Glucose permanently changes the hemoglobin molecule within red blood cells
D. Abnormal fat levels in the blood
E. Formation of plaque along the inside walls of blood vessels
F. Sugars and starches
G. Sugar in the urine
H. Cholesterol derived from the diet
I. Man-made hydrogenated fats
J. Elevated blood sugar
K. Fats and proteins that are able to convert to glucose if necessary
L. Electrolytes consisting of positively or negatively charged particles
M. Excessively high blood insulin levels
N. Hormone produced by the pancreas to lower blood glucose
O. Diagnosis based on the patient's initial signs and symptoms
P. Excessive fat in blood, giving a milky appearance in the plasma
Q. Condition of excessive ketones in the blood causing an acid condition
R. Hormone produced by the pancreas to raise blood glucose
S. Stored form of glucose especially found in muscles and the liver
T. Cholesterol manufactured in the liver
U. Final, confirmed diagnosis based on clinical signs and symptoms and the results of diagnostic tests

FUNDAMENTAL CONCEPTS

22. Provide the missing information in the plasma flow chart (see Figure 6-1 in the textbook).

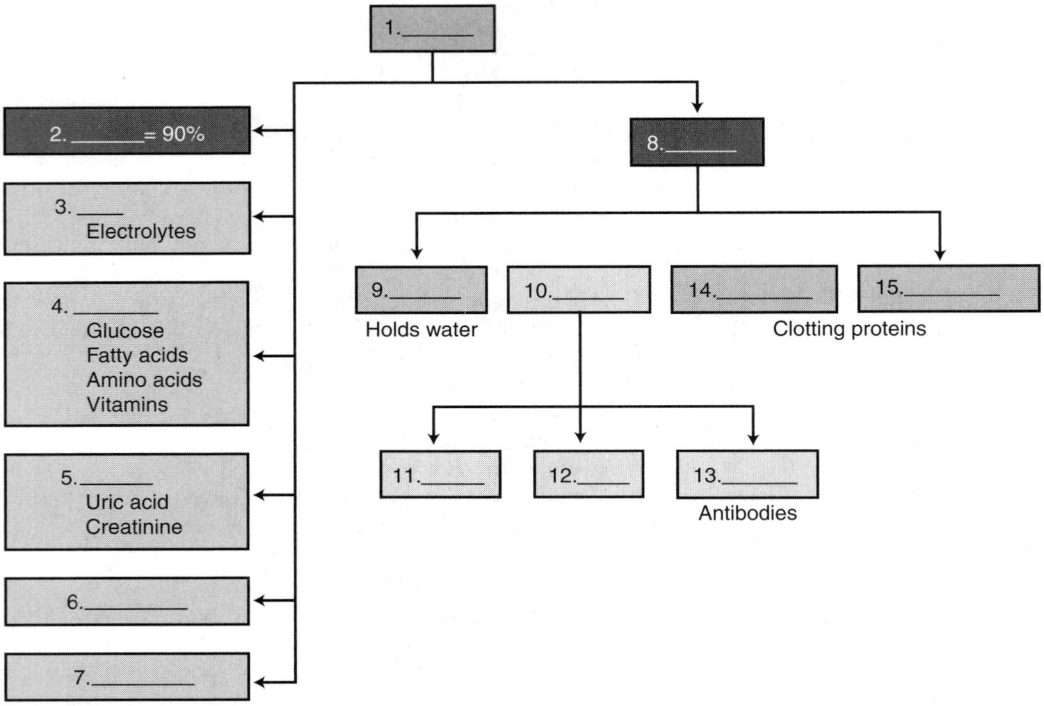

23. Match the categories of chemicals found in plasma with their associated substances (see Figure 6-1 in the textbook).

_______ clotting proteins
_______ nutrients
_______ hormones
_______ proteins
_______ wastes
_______ salts
_______ gamma globulins
_______ enzymes
_______ the three globulins

A. Albumins and globulins
B. Electrolytes
C. Alpha, beta, and gamma
D. Catalysts
E. Glucose, amino acids, and fatty acids
F. Antibodies
G. Thyroid and pituitary glands
H. Prothrombin and fibrinogen
I. Urea, uric acid, creatinine

24. Describe the similarities and differences between the gold "SST" tube and the red "clot" tube.

____

____

____

25. Refer to the sample requisition in the textbook (see Figure 6-3), and identify what tube to use for each of the following tests:

prothrombin time	____________	BUN	____________
lipid panel	____________	CBC w/Diff	____________
renal function panel	____________	mono test	____________

26. When prothrombin and fibrinogen are removed from plasma, the remaining liquid is referred to as ______________________________.

27. Define the following glucose-related abbreviations.

A1c	______________________________	IGT	______________________________
FBG	______________________________	NIDDM	______________________________
FPG	______________________________	OGTT	______________________________
GTT	______________________________	2-hr PP	______________________________
IDDM	______________________________		

28. How is glucose metabolized in the following locations?

Body cells ____

Liver ____

Muscles ____

Adipose tissue ____

29. List the two ways insulin lowers the level of blood glucose.

____

____

30. List the two ways glucagon raises the level of blood glucose.

____

____

31. What two lifestyle changes can a prediabetic patient make to prevent or delay the development of type 2 diabetes?

____

____

32. List three beneficial functions of cholesterol.

____

____

____

33. List the two dietary fats that elevate the bad type of cholesterol (LDL).

____

____

34. Define the following lipid-related abbreviations.

HDL ____________________

LDL ____________________

TC/HDL ratio ____________________

VLDL ____________________

35. List two dietary fats that elevate the good type of cholesterol (HDL).

____

____

36. Why is LDL cholesterol referred to as "lousy" cholesterol and HDL referred to as "healthy" cholesterol?

____

____

37. Physicians are likely to be more interested in which of the following as a predictive indicator of future myocardial infarction?
   a. Cholesterol value
   b. LDL value
   c. Cholesterol/HDL ratio
   d. HDL value

38. People who exercise regularly, maintain normal weight, and eat mostly unsaturated fats will probably increase their level of
   a. HDL
   b. LDL
   c. Albumin
   d. Glucose

39. When testing for triglycerides, the patient should refrain from alcohol for ________ days before testing and fast for ________ hours before the test.

PROCEDURES: CLINICAL LABORATORY IMPROVEMENT AMENDMENT (CLIA)–WAIVED CHEMISTRY TESTS

40. What is the purpose of *calibrating* a blood chemistry analyzer? (Hint: Think of the calibrator checks when running the Cholestech.)

____

____

41. Complete the following tasks.

A. List three reasons or causes why a liquid control would fall outside its designated range.

____

____

____

B. Using the monthly Levy-Jennings chart at the end of this chapter, record the following control settings and daily results for the normal liquid glucose control:

Reference range for control = 96 – 136 mg/dL

+2 standard deviations = 136

+1 standard deviation = 126

Mean = 116

– 1 standard deviation = 106

–2 standard deviations = 96

Daily results:

1. 118	7. 108	13. 137	17. repeat 110	23. 120	29. 114
2. 114	8. 114	13. repeat 125	18. 99	24. 114	30. 115
3. 113	9. 120	14. 117	19. 105	25. 133	31. 116
4. 104	10. 118	15. 106	20. 105	26. 123	
5. 101	11. 120	16. 114	21. 110	27. 130	
6. 100	12. 130	17. 94	22. 118	28. 116	

C. When looking at the chart, were any of the Westgard Rules below broken (circle the numbers that apply)? Should you continue using the monitor and/or strips? ________:

1. Both levels of control results were outside the manufacturer's reference range (if running a normal and high control). *Note:* This rule does not apply because we are monitoring only one control.
2. The same control level fell outside of the reference range in two successive runs.
3. One of the controls fell outside of the plus or minus 1 standard deviation in four successive runs.
4. One of the controls consistently fell above the mean value or consistently fell below the mean value for 10 consecutive runs.

D. (OPTIONAL) If available, chart the class results for the liquid glucose control on the Levy-Jennings chart found in the workbook Appendix, and analyze the results based on the Westgard Rules.

42. List three foods that the patient should avoid 2 days before collecting a fecal specimen used for the occult blood test.

____

____

43. What is the name of home fecal occult blood test for which the patient places the test paper directly into the toilet? ________ If the test area of the paper turns green or blue, is the result positive or negative? ________

44. Label the supplies and equipment for the test kit method for A1c (see Procedure 6-2 in the textbook). Which supply item must be used for all 20 tests in the kit? ________. May that item be used with cartridges from another kit? ________

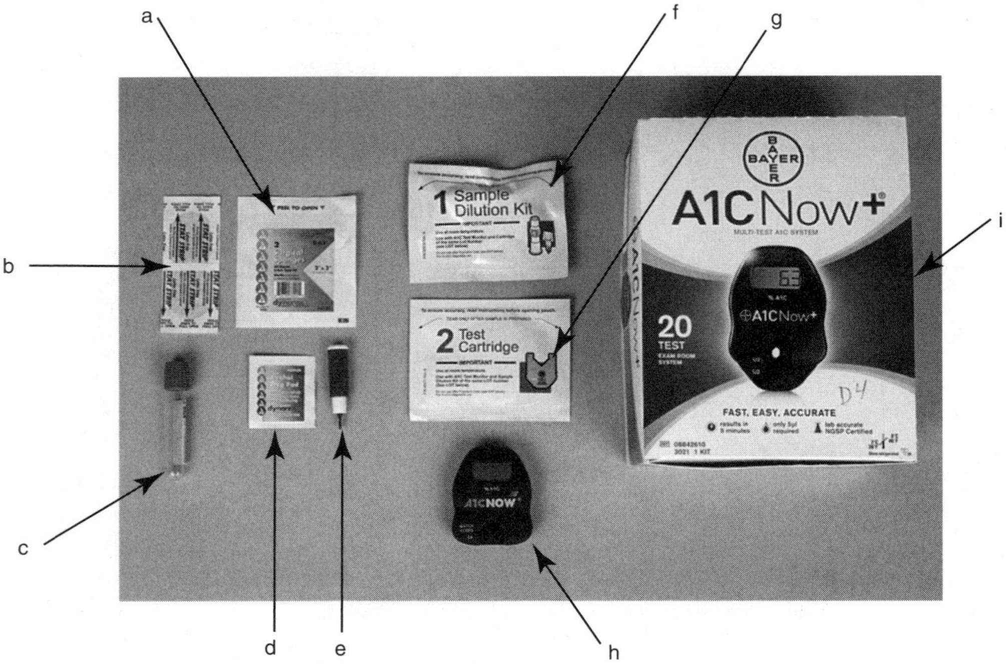

45. Label the Cholestech LDX equipment and supplies (see Procedure 6-3 in the textbook).

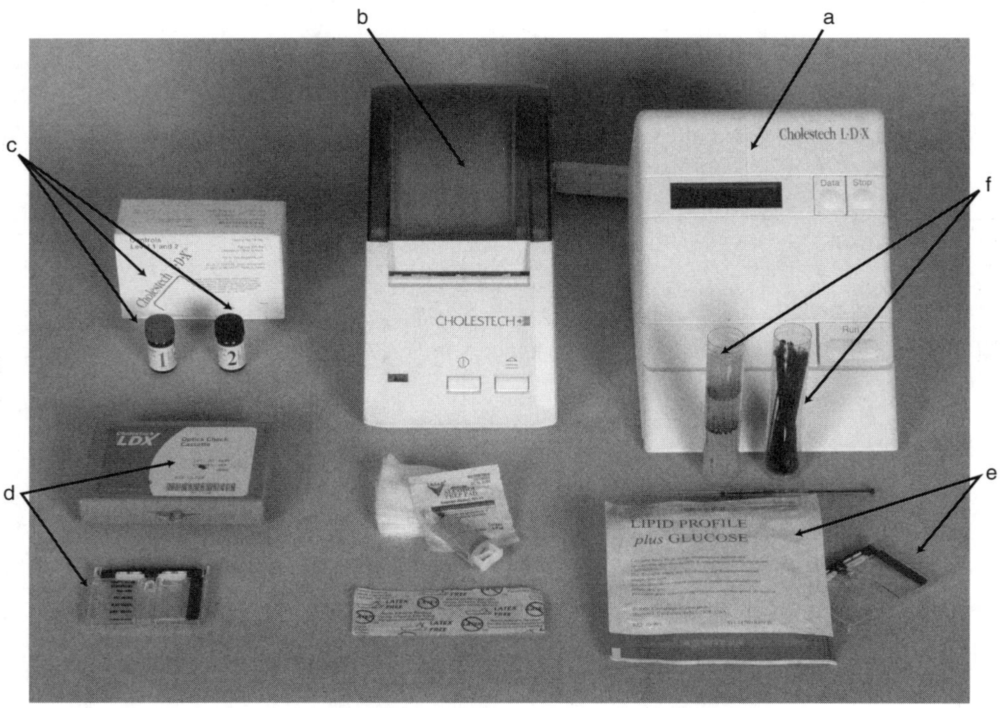

46. Label the ColoScreen III equipment and supplies (see Procedure 6-4 in the textbook).

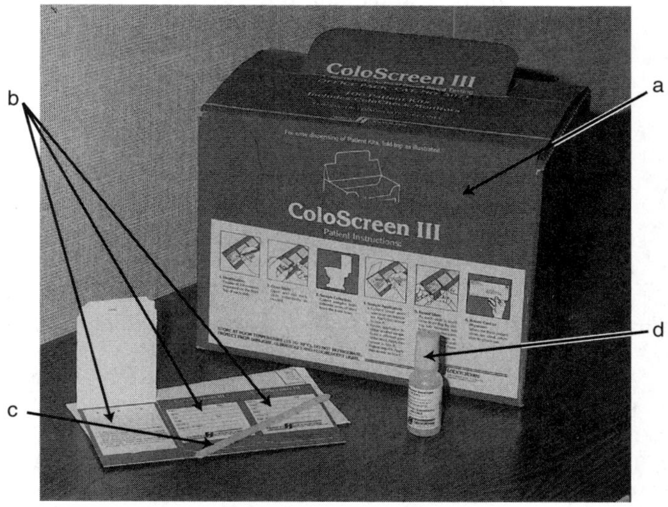

ADVANCED CONCEPTS

Match each procedural and advanced term with the correct definition.

_______ 47. cation
_______ 48. galvanometer
_______ 49. reflectance photometry
_______ 50. troponins I and T
_______ 51. bilirubin
_______ 52. absorbance photometry
_______ 53. anion
_______ 54. i-STAT and Piccolo
_______ 55. transmittance photometry
_______ 56. calibration
_______ 57. occult
_______ 58. gout
_______ 59. myoglobin

A. Form of arthritis caused by accumulation of uric acid crystals in the synovial fluid
B. Hidden or not visible to the naked eye
C. Heme-containing, oxygen-binding protein found in muscles
D. Positively charged ion
E. "Optics check" or setting to ensure the analyzer's optics are working correctly with the testing devices
F. Measurement of the amount of light passing through the solution
G. CLIA-waived chemistry analyzers
H. Heart-specific indicators of a recent myocardial infarction
I. Measurement of the light that reflects off of the specimen
J. Measurement of the amount of light the solution absorbs
K. Waste product from the breakdown of hemoglobin
L. Negatively charged ion
M. Instrument capable of measuring the intensity of light

60. List eight critical chemistry tests that are typically monitored during a medical emergency:

_______________ _______________
_______________ _______________
_______________ _______________
_______________ _______________

61. Match the panels with their representative group of tests.

_______ cardiac panel
_______ hepatic panel
_______ renal panel
_______ lipid panel
_______ thyroid panel
_______ metabolic panel
_______ electrolyte panel

A. Twelve or more tests
B. BUN, creatinine, uric acid
C. Sodium, potassium, chloride
D. Bilirubin, AST, ALT, ALP, LD, GGT
E. Troponins I and T, CK, LD, ALT, myoglobin
F. TSH, T_4, T_3 uptake
G. TC, HDL, LDL, triglycerides

62. Match the analytes with the medical condition or organ that is being monitored.

_______ uric acid
_______ cholesterol
_______ BUN
_______ glucose
_______ bilirubin

A. Diabetes
B. Hepatitis or liver function
C. Gout
D. Coronary artery disease and atherosclerosis
E. Nephritis or kidney function

Chemistry Abbreviations

63. Using the alphabetical list of abbreviations at the beginning of Chapter 6 in the textbook, identify the six enzyme abbreviations routinely tested for tissue or organ damage. (Hint: Remember enzymes have the suffix *-ase*.) Then identify two organs or the diseases that are associated with each enzyme. Use the categorical chart of blood chemistry analytes (see Table 6-3 in the textbook) at the end of the chapter to locate the diseases.

Enzyme Abbreviation	Enzyme	Affected Organs and Associated Diseases
1.		
2.		
3.		
4.		
5.		
6.		

64. List the four electrolyte abbreviations found at the beginning of the chapter and state whether they are cations or anions. (Hint: They have positive or negative charges after their abbreviations.)

Electrolyte Abbreviation	Electrolyte	Cation/Anion (+/–)
1.		
2.		
3.		
4.		

Procedure 6-1: Glucometer Procedure

Person evaluated ______________________ Date ______________________

Evaluated by ______________________ Score ______________________

Outcome goal	To perform FDA-approved CLIA-waived glucose test following the most current OSHA safety guidelines and applying correct quality control
Conditions	Supplies needed: - CONTOUR monitor (previously Ascensia Elite) or One Touch Test Strips - Coded test strip and liquid control - Lancet, alcohol, gauze, bandage - Personal protective equipment
Standards	Required time = 5 minutes Performance time ____________ Total possible points = ____________ Points earned = ____________
Evaluation Rubric Codes: **S** = Satisfactory, meets standard **U** = Unsatisfactory, fails to meet standard	
NOTE: Steps marked with an asterisk (*) are critical to achieve required competency	

Preparation	**Scores**	
	S	**U**
A. Test information		
- Kit or instrument method: **Contour or One Touch Ultra**		
- Manufacturer: **Bayer or LifeScan**		
- Proper storage (e.g., temperature, light) **test strips and controls are stored at room temperature**		
- Expiration date: ______________________		
- Lot #: ______________ Calibration # ______________		
- Package insert or test flow chart available: ________ yes ________ no		
B. Personal protective equipment: **gloves, gown, biohazard container**		
C. Specimen information		
- Type of specimen: **fasting, 2-hour postprandial, or random specimen**		
- Specimen source: **capillary blood or lavender-topped vacuum tube** (Note: gray-topped tubes are not used for this method.)		
- Specimen testing device: **coded test strips**		
D. Assembled all the above, sanitized hands, and applied personal protective equipment.		

Procedure: Analytical Phase	Scores S	Scores U
E. Performed/observed quantitative quality control		
- Calibration check is done automatically when each strip is inserted.		
- (*Note:* Older versions need to set the code number on the meter based on the test strip number,)		
- Control levels: normal ________ high ________		
- (Manufacturer recommendation: Run normal control with each new batch of strips, with each new operator, and then weekly.)		
F. Performed patient test		
1. Turned on meter by inserting test strip's end with the contact bars.		
2. Stuck finger and *touched the end of the strip into the drop* of blood, allowing the blood to flow ("sip") into the strip without interruption.		
- Did **not** smear or place blood on top or bottom of strip.		
3. When beep was heard, removed the glucometer and strip away from drop of blood.		
4. Result displayed on the screen.		
***Accurate Results** ____________ **Instructor Confirmation** ____________		

Follow-up: Postanalytical Phase	Scores S	Scores U
*G. Proper documentation		
1. On control log: ________ yes ________ no		
2. On patient log: ________ yes ________ no		
3. Documentation on patient chart (see following page)		
H. Identified "critical values" and took appropriate steps to notify physician		
- Expected ranges for glucose based on ADA recommendations		

	Fasting	2-Hour Postprandial (After Drinking a Glucose-Rich Beverage)
Normal	Less than 100 mg/dL	<140 mg/dL
Prediabetes	100-125 mg/dL	140-199 mg/dL
Diabetes	≥126 mg/dL	≥200 mg/dL

	S	U
I. Proper disposal and disinfection		
1. Disposed all sharps into biohazard sharps containers.		
2. Disposed all other regulated medical waste into biohazard bags.		
3. Disinfected test area and instruments according to OSHA guidelines.		
4. Sanitized hands after removing gloves.		
Total Points per Column		

Patient Name: ______________________

Patient Chart Entry: (Include when, what, how, why, any additional information, and the signature of the person charting.)

____

____

____

____

Procedure 6-2: A1c NOW+ Glycosylated Hemoglobin Procedure

Person evaluated ______________________ Date ______________

Evaluated by ______________________ Score ______________

Outcome goal	To perform FDA-approved glycosylated hemoglobin A_{1c} waived test following the most current OSHA safety guidelines and applying the correct quality control
Conditions	Supplies needed: - Gauze, bandage, alcohol swab - Lancet for capillary blood sample or heparin tube with venous blood sample - Sample dilution kit containing capillary tube collector and sampler body - Test cartridge - A_{1c} monitor programmed to work only with the 20 cartridges in the kit - Personal protective equipment
Standards	Required time = 5 minutes Performance time = ____________ Total possible points = ____________ Points earned = ____________
Evaluation Rubric Codes: **S** = Satisfactory, meets standard **U** = Unsatisfactory, fails to meet standard	
NOTE: Steps marked with an asterisk (*) are critical to achieve required competency.	

Preparation: Preanalytical Phase	Scores	
	S	**U**
A. Test information		
- Kit or instrument method: **A1c NOW+ test kit method.**		
- Manufacturer: **Bayer.**		
- Proper storage (e.g., temperature, light): **Foil-wrapped cartridges and kits are refrigerated. Allow one hour to warm to room temperature.**		
- Expiration date: ______________________		
- Lot # of cartridges: ______________________		
- Package insert or test flow chart available: ________ yes ________ no		
B. Personal protective equipment: **gloves, gown, face shield.**		
C. Proper specimen used for test.		
- Use only **fresh capillary blood** or venous whole blood collected in a **green heparin tube.** Venous blood can be used only if the tube is less than 1 week old and has been refrigerated during that time. Make sure blood in heparin tube is well mixed and at room temperature.		
- Specimen testing device: microcapillary tube provided in kit. After the glass capillary tube has been filled with the specimen, the analysis must begin within 5 minutes.		
D. Assembled all the above and made sure they were at the same temperature (within 18 to 28 degrees Centigrade), sanitized hands, and applied personal protective equipment.		

Procedure: Analytical Phase	Scores S	Scores U
E. Performed/observed quantitative quality control		
- Optics check: Each box of test kits has already set its optics (make sure code on cartridge matches the code on monitor, but do not open until just before inserting into monitor).		
- Control levels: normal ____________ abnormal ____________		
F. Performed patient test		
1. Removed the blood collector from the foil #1 sampler dilution kit, and gently touched the tip of the capillary tube that was attached to the holder into the small drop of blood from the fingerstick or the venous blood drop on the slide.		
- The blood should fill the small glass capillary tube without touching the plastic holder.		
2. Wiped the sides of the capillary tube with tissue.		
3. Fully inserted the capillary holder into the sampler body that also came from the #1 sampler dilution kit (pushed together and twisted until the holder and sampler body snapped into place).		
4. Mixed sample with the dilution by tilting 6 to 8 times; then stood the sampler on the table.		
5. Opened the #2 test cartridge foil package and performed the following within 2 minutes:		
- Clicked the cartridge into the monitor that came in the same kit box; checked code numbers, which must match		
- While the monitor indicated "WAIT," prepared the sample by removing the base		
- Did not add the sample until the monitor indicated "SMPL"		
- Pushed sampler down onto the white well of the cartridge		
- The monitor was on a level surface and was not moved until the test was complete.		
6. After several minutes, the monitor indicated "QCOK," followed by the test result and by the number of tests left in the kit.		
7. Recorded the results from the display and reported to the physician.		
***Accurate Results** ____________ **Instructor Confirmation** ____________		

Follow-up: Postanalytical Phase	Scores S	Scores U
*G. Proper documentation		
1. Control logs: ____________ yes ____________ no		
2. Patient log: ____________ yes ____________ no		
3. Documented on patient chart (see following page).		

4. Identified critical values and took appropriate steps to notify physician.		
- Expected values: Nondiabetics: 3%-6% Controlled diabetics: 6%-8% Poorly controlled diabetics: As much as 20% or higher *Note:* Because A_{1c} is also affected by the hemoglobin concentration, normal ranges should be determined by each laboratory to conform to the population being tested.		
H. Proper disposal and disinfection		
1. Disposed the cartridge into biohazard sharps containers, and returned monitor to the box for subsequent testing.		
2. Disposed all other regulated medical waste into biohazard bags.		
3. Disinfected test area and instruments according to OSHA guidelines.		
4. Sanitized hands after removing gloves.		
Total Points per Column		

Patient Name: ______________________________

Patient Chart Entry: (Include when, what, how, why, any additional information, and the signature of the person charting.)

____

____

____

____

Procedure 6-3: Cholestech Method of Measuring Lipids and Glucose

Person evaluated ______________________ Date ______________

Evaluated by ______________________ Score ______________

Outcome goal	To perform FDA-approved lipid profile waived test following the most current OSHA safety guidelines and applying the correct quality control.
Conditions	Supplies needed: - Optics check cassette - Level 1 and 2 liquid controls - Alcohol, gauze, and lancets or vacuum lithium heparin tubes - Capillary tubes and plungers for finger stick sample - Mini-Pet pipette and pipette tips for venipuncture sample - Personal protective equipment
Standards	Required time = 10 minutes Performance time = ____________ Total possible points = ____________ Points earned = ____________
Evaluation Rubric Codes: **S** = Satisfactory, meets standard **U** = Unsatisfactory, fails to meet standard	
NOTE: Steps marked with an asterisk (*) are critical to achieve required competency.	

Preparation: Preanalytical Phase	Scores S	Scores U
A. Test information		
- Kit or instrument method: **Cholestech LDX Analyzer**		
- Manufacturer: **Cholestech Corporation**		
- Proper storage (e.g., temperature, light): **Foil-wrapped cassettes are refrigerated. They must return to room temperature before testing.**		
- Expiration date: ____________		
- Cassette lot #: ____________		
- Package insert or test flow chart available: ________ yes ________ no		
B. Personal protective equipment: **gloves, gown, biohazard containers**		
C. Specimen Information		
- Patient preparation: **Fasting recommended for cholesterol. Triglyceride requires fasting and no alcohol consumption in previous 48 hours.**		
- Type of specimen: **capillary blood or lithium heparin (green) tube only for venous blood**		
- Specimen testing device: **Cholestech capillary tube (once in tube, must be tested within 5 minutes)**		
D. Assembled all the above, sanitized hands, and applied personal protective equipment.		

Procedure: Analytical Phase	Scores	
	S	U
E. Performed/observed quantitative quality control		
- Calibration check: **Run calibration cassette daily.**		
- Control levels: **Level 1, Level 2** (Use the mini-Pet pipettes provided by Cholestech)		
F. Performed patient test	S	U
1. Allowed cassette to come to room temperature (at least 10 minutes before opening).		
2. Made sure analyzer was plugged in and warmed up.		
3. Removed cassette from its pouch and placed it on flat surface.		
- Held cassette by the short sides only.		
- Did not touch the black bar or the brown magnetic strip.		
4. Pressed RUN; the analyzer did a self-test, and the screen displayed "selftest running" and then "selftest OK."		
5. The cassette drawer opened, and the screen displayed "load cassette and press RUN."		
- Drawer remains open for 4 minutes, after which it closes with the message "System timeout: RUN to continue." If the RUN button is not pushed within 15 seconds, the drawer closes, and the screen goes blank. Press RUN again, allow to go through the self-test again, and then proceed.		
6. Collected fresh capillary blood to the black line of the capillary tube with plunger inserted into the red end of the tube.		
- Or collected fresh venous whole blood with the Cholestech mini-Pet pipette.		
7. Placed whole blood sample into the test cassette sample well.		
- The finger stick sample must be put into the cassette within 5 minutes of collection or the blood will clot.		
8. *Immediately* placed cassette into the drawer of the analyzer.		
- Kept cassette level after the sample was applied.		
- The black reaction bar faced toward the analyzer.		
- The brown magnetic strip was on the right.		
9. Pressed RUN. The drawer closed, and the screen displayed "[test names] – running."		
10. When the test was completed, the analyzer beeped, and the screen displayed results at the same time the printer printed results. (Press DATA to display the calculated results of all tests on the screen if running a panel of tests.)		
***Accurate Results** ___________ **Instructor Confirmation** ___________		

Follow-up: Postanalytical Phase	Scores	
	S	U
*G. Proper documentation		
1. On control log: ___________ yes ___________ no		

2. On patient log: ___________ yes ___________ no		
3. Documented on patient chart (see below).		
4. Identified "critical values" and took appropriate steps to notify physician.		
- NCEP ATP III guidelines for lipid panels:		
Test	**Desirable**	
Total cholesterol (TC)	<200 mg/dL	
HDL cholesterol	>40 mg/dL	
LDL cholesterol	<130 mg/dL	
Triglycerides	<150 mg/dL	
TC/HDL ratio	≤4.5	
Glucose	Fasting: 60-110 mg/dL	
	Nonfasting: <less than 160 mg/dL	
Alanine aminotransferase	10-40 U/L	
H. Proper disposal and disinfection		
1. Disposed all sharps into biohazard sharps containers.		
2. Disposed all other regulated medical waste into biohazard bags.		
3. Disinfected test area and instruments according to OSHA guidelines.		
4. Sanitized hands after removing gloves.		
Total Points per Column		

Patient Name: ______________________________

Attach printed readout, or record results on the chart provided:

Test	Results	Desirable
Total cholesterol (TC)		<200 mg/dL
HDL cholesterol		40 mg/dL
LDL cholesterol		<130 mg/dL
Triglycerides		<150 mg/dL
TC/HDL ratio		≤4.5
Other		
Glucose		Fasting: 60-110 mg/dL
		Nonfasting: <160 mg/dL

Procedure 6-4: Occult Blood: ColoScreen III Method

Person evaluated ______________________ Date ______________________

Evaluated by ______________________ Score ______________________

Outcome goal	To perform FDA-approved, CLIA-waived fecal occult blood test following the most current OSHA safety guidelines and applying the correct quality control
Conditions	Supplies needed: - Three specimen slides - Three wooden applicators - Hydrogen peroxide developer - Personal protective equipment
Standards	Required time = 5 minutes Performance time = __________ Total possible points = __________ Points earned = __________
Evaluation Rubric Codes: **S** = Satisfactory, meets standard **U** = Unsatisfactory, fails to meet standard	
NOTE: Steps marked with an asterisk (*) are critical to achieve required competency.	

Preparation: Preanalytical Phase	Scores	
	S	**U**
A. Test information		
- Kit or instrument method: **ColoScreen III**		
- Manufacturer: **SmithKline Diagnostics**		
- Proper storage (e.g., temperature, light): **room temperature**		
- Expiration date: ______________________		
- Lot # on kit: ______________________		
- Package insert or test flow chart available: __________ yes __________ no		
B. Instructed patient on the following dietary preparations.		
1. Two days before the test and during testing time, the patient should eat a high-fiber diet with any of the following:		
- Well-cooked poultry and fish		
- Cooked fruits and vegetables		
- Bran cereals		
- Raw lettuce, carrots, and celery		
- Moderate amounts of peanuts and popcorn		
2. The patient should avoid ingesting the following substances, which interfere with the test results:		
- Red and partially cooked meats		

	S	U
- Turnips, cauliflower, broccoli, parsnips, and melons (especially cantaloupe)		
- Alcohol, aspirin, and vitamin C		
C. Instructed the patient on how to use the slides, applicators, and the take-home instructions as follows:		
- After a bowel movement, use the wooden applicator to collect a small sample of feces, and spread a thin layer in box A of the slide.		
- Using the same applicator, collect a second sample from a different part of the feces, and spread it in box B.		
- Discard the wooden applicator, reseal the cover of the slide, and complete the information requested on the outside of the cover.		
- Repeat above steps with the remaining applicators for the next two bowel movements and two remaining slides.		

Procedure: Analytical Phase	**Scores**	
	S	**U**
D. Personal protective equipment: gloves when testing the slides		
E. Performed occult blood test as follows:		
- Confirmed all necessary information was written on slide covers.		
- Applied gloves and observed universal precautions.		
- Opened the back sides of all three slides and placed two drops of developer on each specimen.		
- Observed slide for 30 seconds to 2 minutes and checked to see if a blue reaction occurred, indicating a positive result.		
F. Performed monitor test (internal control)		
- Placed one or two drops between the monitor boxes and observed for 30 seconds to 2 minutes before reading the results.		
- Confirmed the positive control turned blue and the negative control did not.		
***Accurate Results** ____________ **Instructor Confirmation** ____________		

Follow-up: Postanalytical Phase	**Scores**	
	S	**U**
*G. Proper documentation		
1. On control/patient log: ____________ yes ____________ no		
2. Documented on patient chart (see following page).		
3. Identified critical values and took appropriate steps to notify physician.		
- Expected values for occult blood: negative		
H. Proper disposal and disinfection		
1. Disposed all regulated medical waste into biohazard bags.		
2. Disinfected test area and instruments according to OSHA guidelines.		
3. Sanitized hands after removing gloves.		
Total Points per Column		

Patient Name: ______________________________

Patient Chart Entry: (Include when, what, how, why, any additional information, and the signature of the person charting.)

____

____

____

Procedure 6-5: i-STAT Chemistry Analyzer Procedure

Person evaluated ______________________________ Date ______________________

Evaluated by ______________________________ Score ______________________

Outcome goal	To perform FDA-approved i-STAT chemistry waived test following the most current OSHA safety guidelines and applying the correct quality control
Conditions	Supplies needed: - i-STAT 1 handheld, recharging dock, and printer - Ampule of Level 1 liquid control for i-STAT CHEM 8+ - i-STAT CHEM 8+ cartridges - Fresh blood collected in lithium heparin tubes (green top) - 1-mL plain syringe - Safety transfer device or safety tip - Personal protective equipment and biohazard container
Standards	Required time = 15 minutes Performance time = ____________ Total possible points = ____________ Points earned ____________
Evaluation Rubric Codes: **S** = Satisfactory, meets standard **U** = Unsatisfactory, fails to meet standard	
NOTE: Steps marked with an asterisk (*) are critical to achieve required competency.	

Preparation: Preanalytical Phase	Scores	
	S	**U**
A. Test information		
- Kit or instrument method: **i-STAT Chemistry Analyzer**		
- Manufacturer: **Abbott**		
- Proper storage (e.g., temperature, light): **Foil-wrapped cartridges and controls are refrigerated. They must return to room temperature before testing.**		
- Expiration date: ______________________		
- Scan cartridge lot #: ______________________		
- Package insert or test flow chart available: ________ yes ________ no		
B. Personal protective equipment: **gloves, gown, biohazard containers**		
C. Specimen information		
- Patient preparation: **Collect blood, making sure the 4-mL heparin tube fills completely and is mixed by tilting 10 times. Specimen should be tested within 10 minutes.**		
- Type of specimen: **Lithium heparin (green) tube only for venous blood**		
- Specimen testing device: **A 1-mL syringe is used to remove the specimen from the green vacuum tube and transfer the blood to the cartridge.**		
D. Assembled all the above, sanitized hands, and applied personal protective equipment.		

Procedure: Analytical Phase	Scores S	Scores U
E. Performed/observed quantitative quality control		
- Calibration check: **Use the simulator provided by i-STAT.**		
- Control level: **Level 1 ampule is provided by i-STAT.**		
F. Performed patient test	**S**	**U**
1. Allowed cassette to come to room temperature (at least 10 minutes before opening).		
2. Keyed in operator and patient information into the handheld analyzer, followed by scanning the cartridge bar code until a beep was heard.		
3. *Within 10 minutes* of drawing a 4-mL specimen of blood into a vacuum tube, performed the following:		
- Mixed the specimen by tilting 10 times.		
- Connected a safety tip or safety transfer device to a 1-mL syringe.		
- Inverted the green-top tube with the specimen and pierced the green stopper with the syringe safety tip or the transfer device.		
- *Slowly* pulled back on the syringe plunger until it was about one-half full; noted any air bubbles that entered syringe while transferring and did not push them back into specimen.		
- Disconnected syringe from vacuum tube and continued to hold it with tip pointed upward; then held a gauze pad at tip to absorb blood while syringe plunger slowly pushed out the air and approximately three drops of blood.		
- Tore open the foiled cartridge pouch and removed the cartridge by holding the sides and placed it on a flat surface.		
- Held the syringe tip directly over sample well and carefully pushed the blood into the cartridge until the blood reached the arrow and there was still blood remaining in the well but not overflowing.		
4. Moved the tab over the well from left to right using one finger; did not press on the beige circle area directly over the well; pushed down on the tab until it snapped into place.		
5. Used the grooved area to the left of the well or the sides of the cartridge to slowly insert it into the analyzer.		
- The handheld first displayed "Identifying Cartridge" and then a time-to-result bar.		
- *Did not* remove cartridge until the "Cartridge Locked" message was removed and results were displayed on screen.		
6. Review results		
- After 2 to 3 minutes, the results appeared on the screen. The "→ Page" command on bottom of the screen indicated more results would appear on a second screen. Pressed the print button to send the results to the printer by wireless transmission or by the docking device USB connection.		
The handheld showed the numerical values and units with the results. It also showed bar graphs with tic marks for reference ranges.		
***Accurate Results** ________________ **Instructor Confirmation** ________________		

Follow-up: Postanalytical Phase	Scores	
	S	U
*G. Proper documentation		
1. On control log: ____________ yes ____________ no		
2. On patient log: ____________ yes ____________ no		
3. Documented on patient chart (see below).		
4. Identified "critical values" and took appropriate steps to notify physician.		
*SEE TABLE OF TEST RANGES BELOW.		
H. Proper disposal and disinfection		
1. Disposed all sharps into biohazard sharps containers.		
2. Disposed all other regulated medical waste into biohazard bags.		
3. Disinfected test area and instruments according to OSHA guidelines.		
4. Sanitized hands after removing gloves.		
Total Points per Column		

Test	Test Symbol	Units	Reportable Range	Reference Range	Results	Critical Low/ High
Sodium	Na	mmol/L	100-180	138-146		
Potassium	K	mmol/L	2.0-9.0	3.5-4.9		
Chloride	Cl	mmol/L	65-140	98-109		
Total carbon dioxide	TCO_2	mmol/L	5-50	24-29		
Ionized calcium	iCa	mmol/L	0.25-2.50	1.12-1.32		
Glucose	Glu	mg/dL	20-700	70-105		
Urea nitrogen	BUN	mg/dL	3-140	8-26		
Creatinine	Crea	mg/dL	0.2-20.0	0.6-1.3		
Hematocrit	Hct	% PCV	10-75	38-51		
Hemoglobin*	Hb	g/dL	3.4-25.5	12-17		
Anion gap*	AnGap	mmol/L	10-99	10-20		

Patient Name: ______________________________________

Attach printed readout, or record results on the chart above.

Levy-Jennings Monthly Graph of Daily ________ Controls

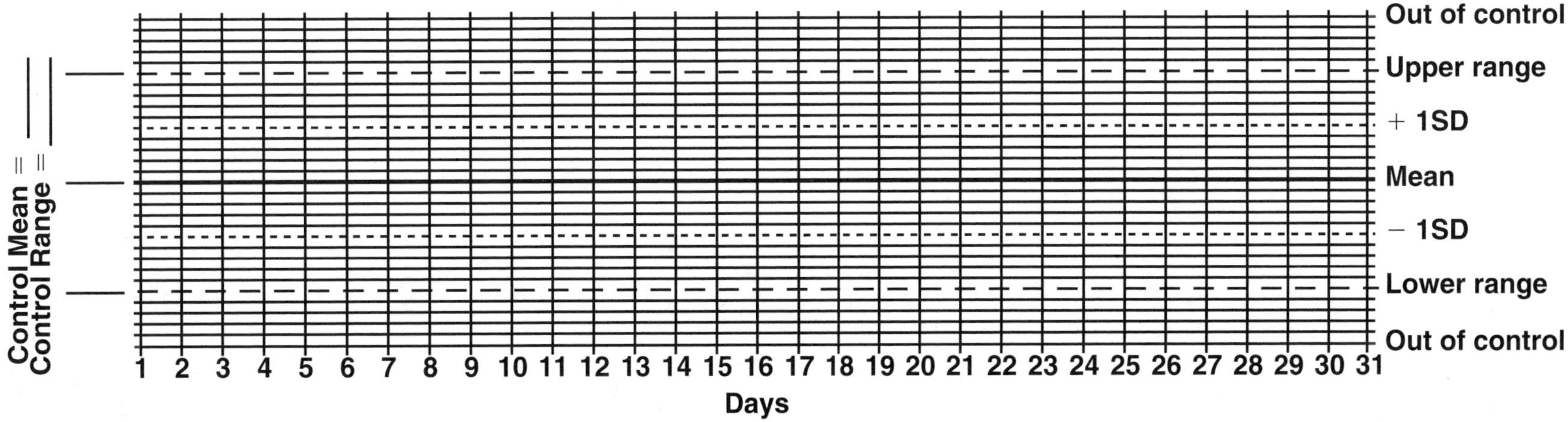

Levy-Jennings Monthly Graph of Daily ________ Controls

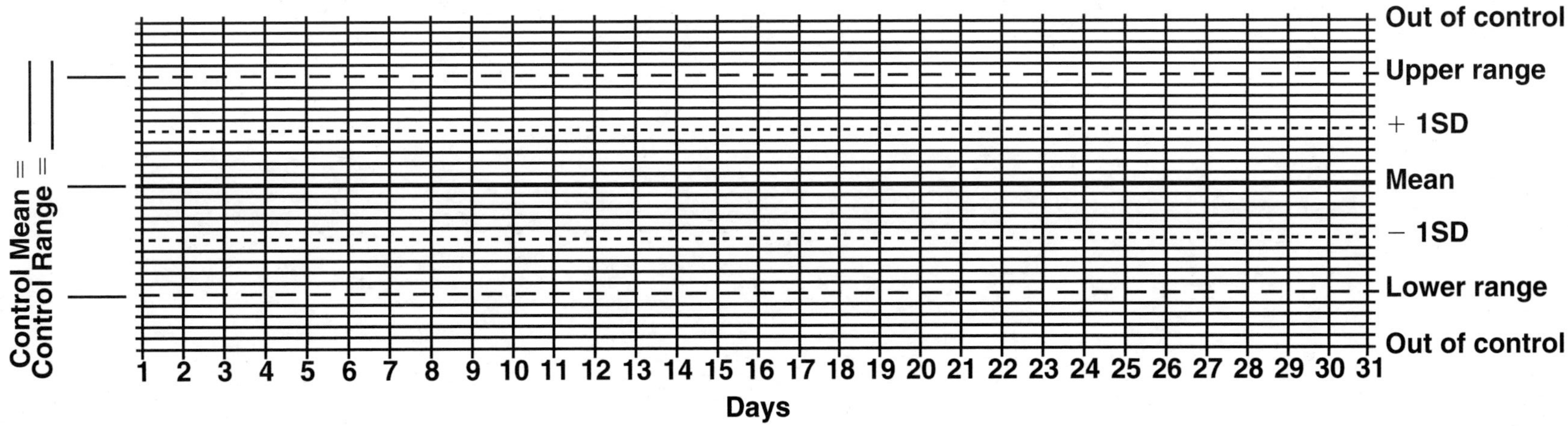

7 Immunology

VOCABULARY REVIEW

Match each term with the correct definition.

A. active immunity
B. autoimmune diseases
C. antibodies
D. antigens
E. cell-mediated immunity
F. complement proteins
G. histamine
H. humoral immunity
I. inflammation
J. interferons
K. mucous membrane
L. natural killer cells
M. normal flora
N. passive immunity
O. phagocytes
P. phagocytosis

________ 1. B lymphocytic cell response to antigens resulting in the production of specific antibodies to destroy a foreign invader; also called antibody-mediated immunity

________ 2. Cells capable of engulfing and ingesting microorganisms and cellular debris

________ 3. Compound released by injured cells that causes the dilation of blood vessels

________ 4. Immunoglobulins produced specifically to destroy foreign invaders

________ 5. Long-term protection against future infections resulting from the production of antibodies formed naturally during an infection or artificially by vaccination

________ 6. Nonpathogenic microorganisms that normally inhabit the skin and mucous membranes

________ 7. Overall reaction of the body to tissue injury or invasion by an infectious agent; characterized by redness, heat, swelling, and pain

________ 8. Process of engulfing and digesting microorganisms and cellular debris

________ 9. Proteins secreted by infected cells to prevent the further replication and spread of an infection into neighboring cells

________ 10. Proteins that stimulate phagocytosis and inflammation and are capable of destroying bacteria

________ 11. Short-term acquired immunity created by antibodies received naturally through the placenta (or the colostrum to an infant) or artificially by injection

________ 12. Special type of lymphocyte that attacks and destroys infected cells and cancer cells in a nonspecific way

________ 13. Substances that are perceived as foreign to the body and elicit an antibody response

________ 14. T-lymphocytic cell response to antigens

________ 15. Thin sheets of tissue that line the internal cavities and canals of the body and serve as a barrier against the entry of pathogens

________ 16. Destructive tissue diseases caused by antibody/self-antigen reactions

Match the B and T lymphocytes with their functions.

A. killer T cells
B. suppressor T cells
C. plasma cells
D. helper T cells (T_H4 or CD4)
E. memory B cells
F. memory T cells

_______ 17. Antigen-activated B lymphocytes that remember an identified antigen for future encounters

_______ 18. Antigen-activated lymphocytes that attack foreign antigens directly and destroy cells that bear the antigens; also called cytotoxic cells

_______ 19. Antigen-activated lymphocytes that inhibit T and B cells after enough cells have been activated

_______ 20. Antigen-activated lymphocytes that stimulate other T cells and help B cells produce antibodies

_______ 21. Antigen-activated T lymphocytes that remember an antigen for future encounters

_______ 22. Subgroup of B lymphocytes that produce the antibodies that travel through the blood specifically targeting and reacting with antigens

Match the immunology testing and disease terms with the correct definition.

A. agglutination	E. immunosorbent	I. serology
B. chromatographic	F. in vitro	J. titer
C. erythroblastosis fetalis	G. in vivo	K. vaccination
D. heterophile antibody	H. self-antigens	L. wheal

_______ 23. Antibody that appears during an Epstein-Barr viral infection (mononucleosis) that has an unusual affinity to heterophile antigens on sheep red cells

_______ 24. Branch of laboratory medicine that performs antibody/antigen testing with serum

_______ 25. Clumping together of blood cells or latex beads caused by antibodies adhering to their antigens

_______ 26. A hemolytic anemia in newborns resulting from maternal-fetal blood group incompatibility

_______ 27. Testing in a laboratory apparatus

_______ 28. Pertaining to a visual color change that appears when an enzyme-linked antibody/antigen reaction occurs

_______ 29. Pertaining to the attachment of an antigen or antibody to a solid surface such as latex beads, wells in plastic dishes, or plastic cartridges

_______ 30. Process of injecting harmless or killed microorganisms into the body to induce immunity against a potential pathogen; also called immunization

_______ 31. Raised induration

_______ 32. Substances within the body that induce the production of antibodies that attack an individual's own body tissues; also called autoantigens

_______ 33. A quantitative test that measures the amount of antibody that reacts with a specific antigen

_______ 34. Testing within a host or living organism

FUNDAMENTAL CONCEPTS

35. When a pathogen is invading the body, list two examples of protection for each line of defense:

    First line of external defenses: ______

    Second line of internal, nonspecific defenses: ______

    ______

    Third line of internal, specific defenses: ______

    ______

36. List two white cells that are phagocytic.

    ______

37. Give an example of a normal flora organism, and describe how it prevents the invasion of pathogens.

    ______

    ______

38. List the clinical signs of inflammation.

    ______

39. Describe antigens.

    ______

    ______

40. Which cells are associated with cell-mediated immunity?

    ______

41. What is another name for antibodies? (Hint: They are a subcategory of proteins.)

    ______

42. Name the five types of antibodies by their immunoglobulin identification.

    ______

43. Refer to Figure 7-4A and B in the textbook and give examples of natural and artificial active immunity and natural and artificial passive immunity.

    ______

    ______

44. The pregnancy test determines the presence of what antigenic substance?

____

____

45. Fill in the blanks for the following medical information regarding infectious mononucleosis:

Causative agent: ______________________

Clinical symptoms: ______________________

Hematology findings: ______________________

Immunology findings: ______________________

46. Label the QuickVue+ infectious mononucleosis supplies (see Procedure 7-2 in the textbook).

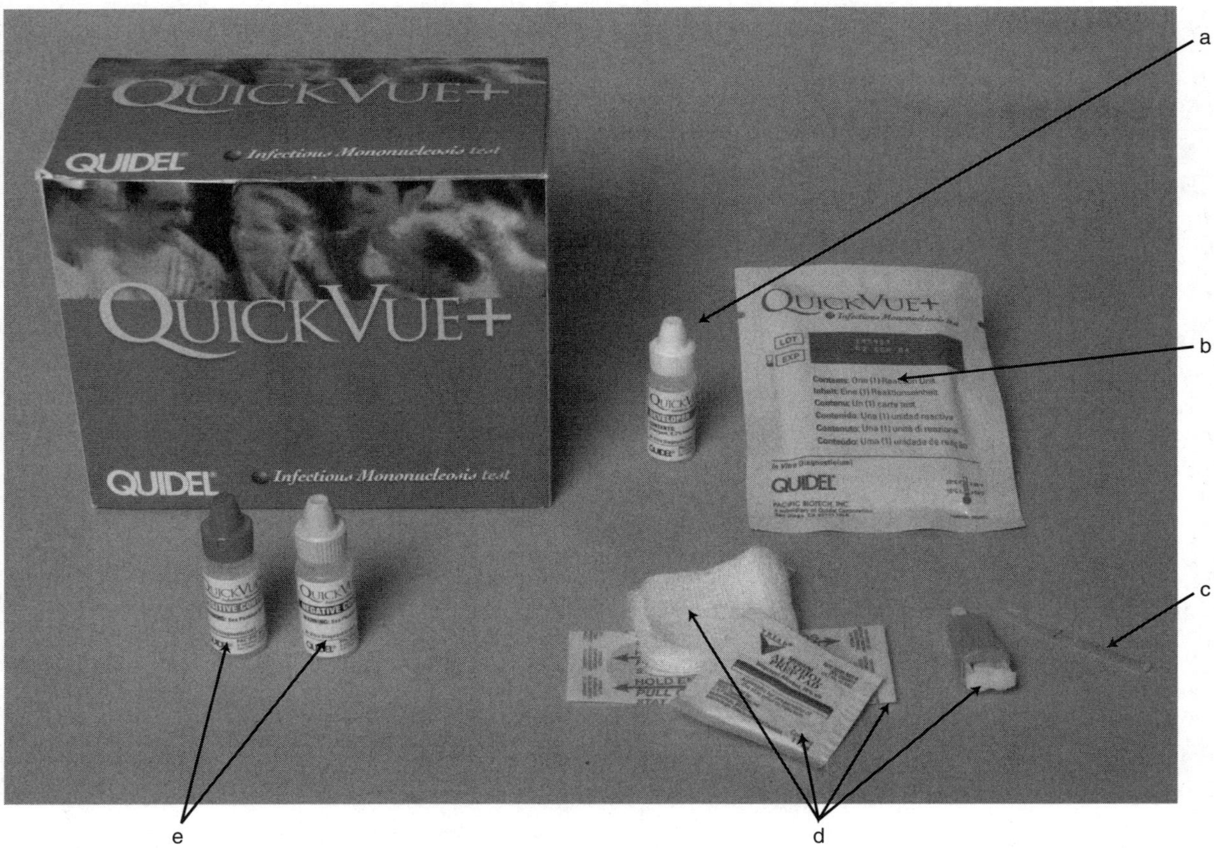

47. Describe the relation between *Helicobacter pylori* and ulcers.

____

____

48. Label the QuickVue *H. pylori* supplies (see Procedure 7-3 in the textbook).

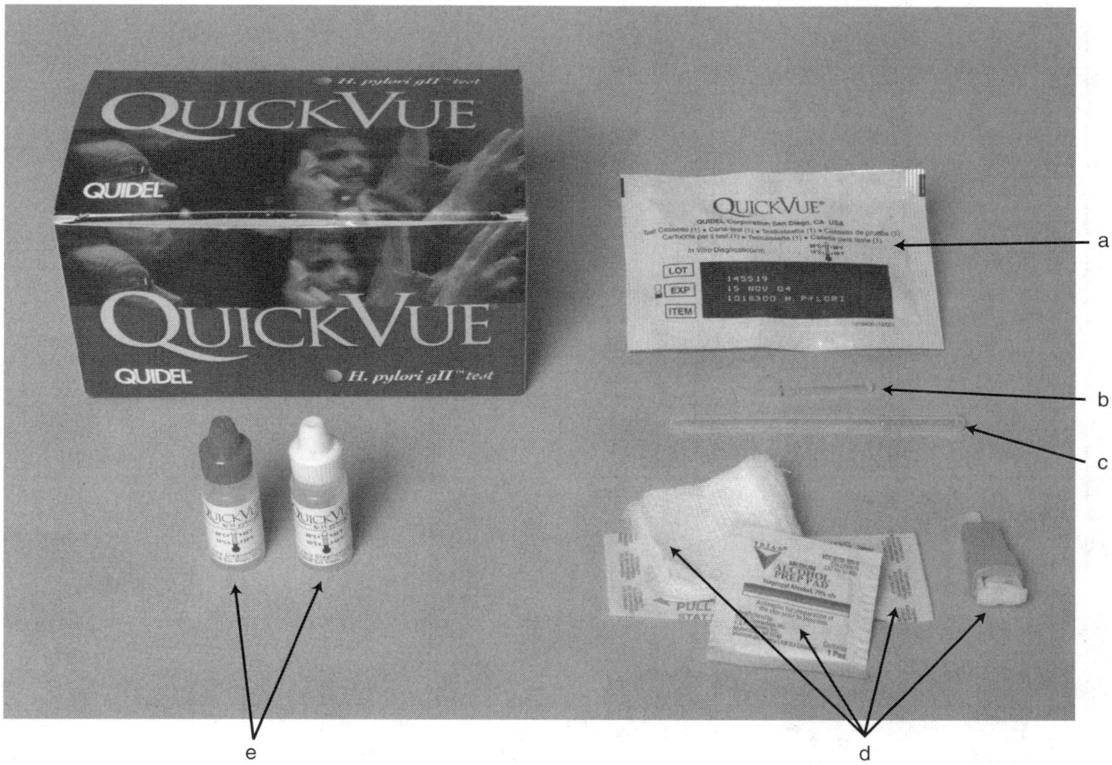

49. Based on the test results illustrated in the chart, interpret the results for each test as negative, positive, or invalid.

<table>
<tr><th></th><th>Test</th><th>Figure in Textbook</th><th>Interpreted Result</th></tr>
<tr><td>A</td><td>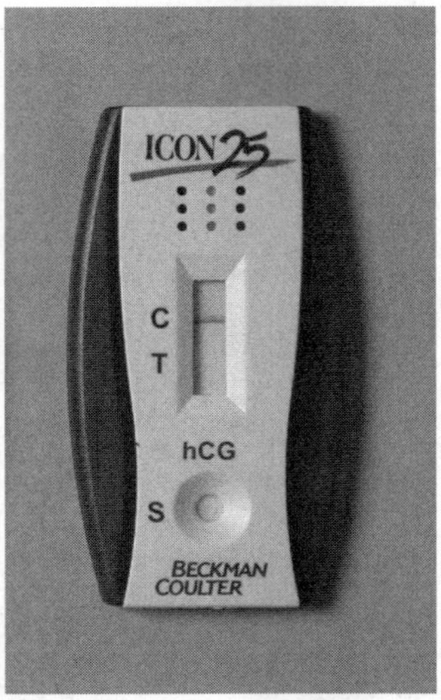
</td><td>Figure 7-6</td><td></td></tr>
<tr><td>B</td><td>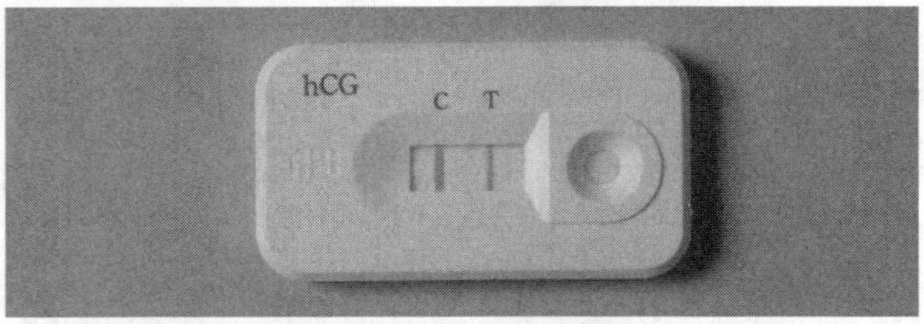
</td><td>Procedure 7-1B</td><td></td></tr>
<tr><td>C</td><td>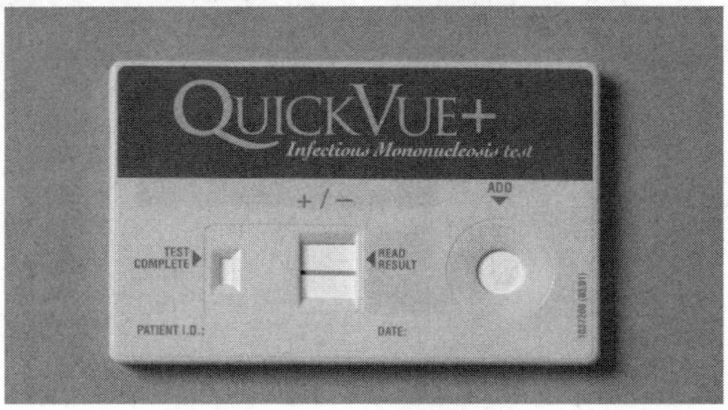
</td><td>Procedure 7-2D</td><td></td></tr>
</table>

50. List three methods for testing for fecal occult blood. (Hint: Two methods are in Chapter 6, and one is in Chapter 7.)

____

____

____

ADVANCED CONCEPTS

51. Define agglutination.

52. Define immunohematology, and give three reasons why testing is done in this area.

53. Name the blood type for a person who has the following: A and D antigens on red blood cells and anti-B antibodies in the serum.

54. Name the antigens and antibodies found in type AB blood.

55. Identify the following ABO blood types based on their agglutination reactions with anti-A and anti-B sera. (Hint: See Procedure 7-4 in the textbook.)

Blood Type	Reaction with Anti-A and Anti-B	
____________		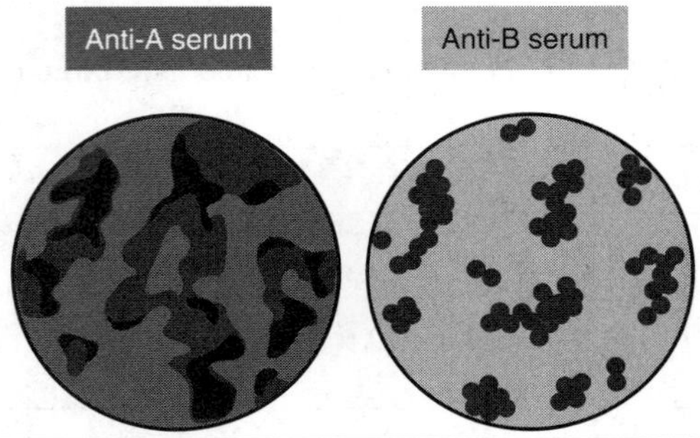
____________		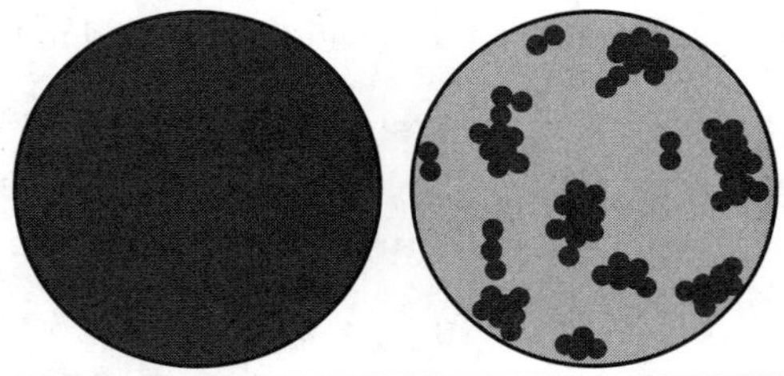
____________		
____________		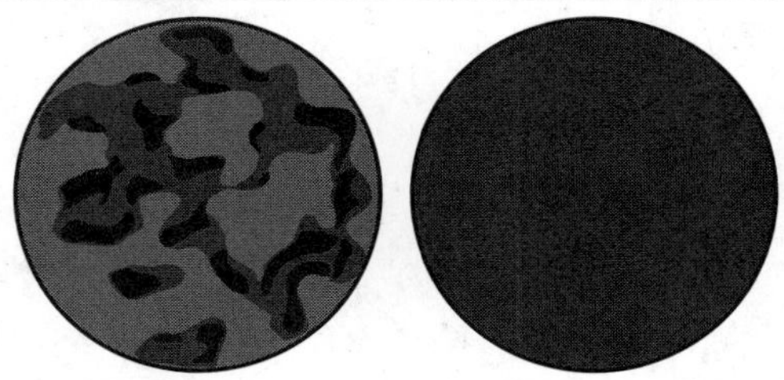

56. Identify which of the following is Rh positive and which is Rh negative. (Hint: See Procedure 7-4 in the textbook.)

Rh Type	Reaction with Rh (anti-D) on the Left and the Negative Control on the Right
________________	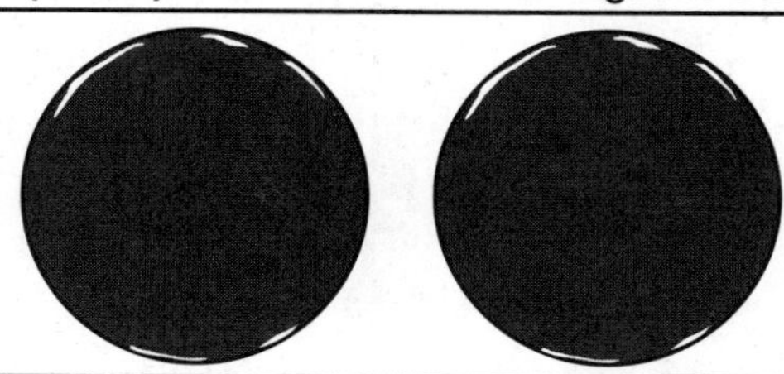
________________	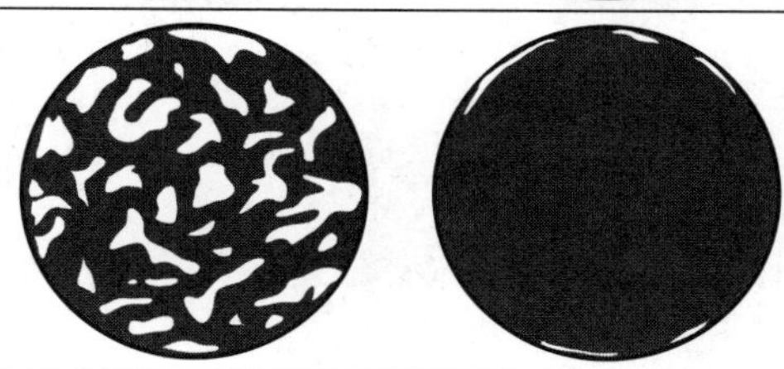

57. When the body is exposed to the following pathogens, it produces specific antibodies that can be measured in the plasma or serum. Refer to Table 7-3 in the textbook, and identify the following pathogenic diseases and indicate whether the pathogen is a bacteria or virus.

Pathogen Disease	Bacteria or Virus
RSV	
Rubella	
Chlamydia	
Varicella zoster	
B. burgdorferi	

58. List three cancers that can be detected by immunologic testing (see Table 7-3 in the textbook).

____

____

Procedure 7-1: SureStep Pregnancy Test Procedure

Person evaluated ______________________ Date ______________

Evaluated by ______________________ Score ______________

Outcome goal	To perform FDA-approved, CLIA-waived urine pregnancy test following the most current OSHA safety guidelines and applying the correct quality control

Conditions	Supplies required:
	- SureStep test kit containing
	  - Individually wrapped test devices
	  - Disposal dropper pipettes
	  - Instruction insert
	- Other materials needed
	  - Urine collection container
	  - Timer
	  - Liquid positive and negative controls for human chorionic gonadotropin (hCG)

Standards	Required time = 5 minutes Performance time = __________ Total possible points = __________ Points earned = __________
Evaluation Rubric Codes: **S** = Satisfactory, meets standard **U** = Unsatisfactory, fails to meet standard	
NOTE: Steps marked with an asterisk (*) are critical to achieve required competency.	

SureStep Pregnancy Test		
Preparation: Preanalytical Phase	**Scores**	
	S	**U**
A. Test information		
- Kit method: **SureStep**		
- Manufacturer: **Applied Biotech, Inc**.		
- Proper storage (e.g., temperature, light): **refrigerator or room temperature**		
- Lot # of kit: ______________________		
- Expiration date: ______________________		
- Package insert or test flow chart available: __________ yes __________ no		
B. Personal protective equipment: **gloves, gown, biohazard container**		
C. Specimen information: **clear urine specimen (centrifuge if cloudy)**		
- Type of specimen: **Preferably first morning urine specimen. Urine can be stored in refrigerator for up to 72 hours but must be tested at room temperature.**		
- Appropriate container: **clean, dry, plastic or glass container**		

Procedure for SureStep hCG: Analytical Phase	Scores S	Scores U
D. Performed/observed qualitative quality control		
- External liquid controls: positive ______________ negative ______________		
- Internal control: **Colored band appears in the control region (C).**		
E. Performed patient test	**S**	**U**
1. Sanitized hands and applied gloves.		
2. Removed test device from its protective pouch and labeled with patient identification.		
- Brought to room temperature before opening to avoid condensation.		
3. Drew up the urine sample to the line marked on the pipette provided in kit.		
- Approximately 0.2 mL		
- Used separate pipettes and devices for each specimen and control.		
4. Dispensed entire contents into the sample well.		
5. Waited for pink-colored bands to appear.		
- High concentrations of hCG can be observed in as little as 40 seconds.		
- Low concentrations may need 4 minutes for the reaction time.		
- Did not interpret results after 10 minutes.		
6. At 5 minutes, read and recorded the results (circled result).		
- Positive = Two distinct pink bands appear, one in the patient test region (T) and one in the control region (C).		
- Negative = Only one pink band appears in the control region (C); no apparent pink band appears in the patient test region (T).		
- Invalid = a total absence of pink bands in control region; test must be repeated with a new device. If problem persisted, called for assistance.		
***Accurate Results** ______________ **Instructor Confirmation** ______________		

Follow-up: Postanalytical	Scores S	Scores U
*F. Proper documentation		
1. On control/patient log: ______________ yes ______________ no		
2. Documented on patient chart (see following page).		
3. Identified critical values and took appropriate steps to notify physician.		
- Expected values for analyte: negative for pregnancy		

G. Proper disposal and disinfection		
1. Disposed all sharps into biohazard sharps containers.		
2. Disposed all other regulated medical waste into biohazard bags.		
3. Disinfected test area and instruments according to OSHA guidelines.		
Total Points per Column		

Patient Name: ____

Patient Chart Entry: (Include when, what, how, why, any additional information, and the signature of the person charting.)

____

____

____

Procedure 7-2: QuickVue+ Mononucleosis Test Procedure

Person evaluated ______________________ Date ______________

Evaluated by ______________________ Score ______________

Outcome goal	To perform FDA-approved, CLIA-waived infectious mononucleosis test following the most current OSHA safety guidelines and applying the correct quality control
Conditions	Supplies required: - QuickVue test kit containing: - Developer - Individually wrapped reaction units - Capillary tubes for capillary blood and pipettes for venous blood - Positive and negative liquid controls - Instruction insert and pictorial flow chart - Other materials needed - Capillary puncture supplies (lancet, alcohol, gauze, bandage), or whole blood venipuncture specimen - Timer - Personal protective equipment
Standards	Required time = 10 minutes Performance time = ___________ Total possible points = ___________ Points earned = ___________
Evaluation Rubric Codes: **S** = Satisfactory, meets standard **U** = Unsatisfactory, fails to meet standard	
NOTE: Steps marked with an asterisk (*) are critical to achieve required competency.	

Preparation for Mononucleosis Test: Preanalytical Phase	Scores	
	S	**U**
A. Test information		
- Kit method: **QuickVue+ Mononucleosis Test**		
- Manufacturer: **Quidel**		
- Proper storage (e.g., temperature, light): **room temperature**		
- Lot # of kit: ______________________		
- Expiration date: ______________________		
- Package insert or test flow chart available ___________ yes ___________ no		
B. Personal protective equipment: **gloves, gown, biohazard containers**		
C. Specimen information		
- Use the capillary transfer tube provided in the kit to obtain capillary blood or the larger transfer pipette in the kit to obtain the venipuncture whole blood and the liquid controls.		

Procedure for Mononucleosis: Analytical Phase	Scores S	Scores U
D. Performed/observed qualitative quality control		
- External liquid controls: positive ______ negative ______		
- Internal control: **The color blue fills the "read result" window.**		
E. Performed patient test	S	U
1. Dispensed all the blood from the capillary tube into the "add" well or transferred a large drop from the venous whole blood specimen with the pipette.		
2. Added five drops of developer to the "add" well.		
- Held bottle vertical and allowed drops to fall freely.		
3. Read results at 5 minutes.		
- "Test complete" line must be visible by 10 minutes.		
4. Interpretation of results (circled result):		
- Positive = Any shade of a blue vertical line forms a positive (+) sign in the "read result" window along with the blue "test complete" line. Even a faint blue vertical line should be reported as a positive result.		
- Negative = No blue vertical line appears in the "read result" window along with the blue "test complete" line.		
- Invalid = After 10 minutes, no signal is observed in the "test complete" window, or the color blue fills the "read result" window. If either occurs, the test must be repeated with a new reaction unit. If the problem continues, contact technical support.		
***Accurate Results** ______ **Instructor Confirmation** ______		

Follow-up: Postanalytical Phase	Scores S	Scores U
*F. Proper documentation		
1. On control/patient log: ______ yes ______ no		
2. Documented on patient chart (see following page).		
3. Identified critical values and took appropriate steps to notify physician.		
- Expected values for analyte: negative for mononucleosis		

G. Proper disposal and disinfection		
1. Disposed all sharps into biohazard sharps containers.		
2. Disposed all other regulated medical waste into biohazard bags.		
3. Disinfected test area and instruments according to OSHA guidelines.		
4. Sanitized hands after removing gloves.		
Total Points per Column		

Patient Name: ____

Patient Chart Entry: (Include when, what, how, why, any additional information, and the signature of the person charting.)

____

____

____

Procedure 7-3: QuickVue *Helicobacter pylori* gII Test (CLIA-Waived) Procedure

Person evaluated ______________________ Date ______________

Evaluated by ______________________ Score ______________

Outcome goal	To perform a CLIA-waived *H. pylori* test following the most current OSHA safety guidelines and applying the correct quality controls
Conditions	Supplies required: - QuickVue *H. pylori* test kit containing - Foil-wrapped test cassettes - Plastic capillary tubes for fingerstick blood - Disposable droppers for venous blood - Liquid controls: positive and negative external controls - Direction insert and procedure card - Other materials needed - Capillary puncture supplies (lancet, alcohol, gauze, bandage) or whole blood venipuncture specimen - Timer - Personal protective equipment
Standards	Required time = 10 minutes Performance time = ______ Total possible points = ______ Points earned = ______
Evaluation Rubric Codes: **S** = Satisfactory, meets standard **U** = Unsatisfactory, fails to meet standard	
NOTE: Steps marked with an asterisk (*) are critical to achieve required competency.	

Preparation for *H. pylori* Test: Preanalytical Phase	**Scores**	
	S	**U**
A. Test information		
- Kit method: **QuickVue *H. pylori* gII test**		
- Manufacturer: **Quidel**		
- Proper storage of kit: **room temperature**		
- Lot # of kit: ______________		
- Expiration date: ______________		
- Package insert or test flow chart available: ______ yes ______ no		
B. Personal protective equipment: gloves, gown, biohazard containers		
C. Specimen information		
- Use the capillary tube provided in the kit to obtain capillary blood or the larger disposable dropper in the kit to obtain the venipuncture whole blood specimen and the liquid controls.		
Procedure for *H. pylori*: Analytical Phase	**Scores**	
	S	**U**
D. Performed/observed qualitative quality control		
- External liquid controls: positive ______ negative ______		
- Internal control: **a blue band of color near the letter C**		

E. Performed patient test	S	U
1. Dispensed the blood into the sample well by one of the following methods:		
- Transferred a large drop from the venous anticoagulated whole blood specimen with the disposable dropper.		
- Dispensed all the finger stick blood from the capillary tube.		
- Added two hanging drops of whole blood directly from a finger stick into the round sample well on the test cassette.		
2. Read and recorded results at 5 minutes.		
- Did not move the test cassette until the assay was complete.		
- Some positive results may be seen earlier than 5 minutes.		
3. Interpretation of results (circle result).		
- Positive = a pink line next to the letter T and a blue line next to the letter C		
- Negative = only a blue line next to the letter C		
- Invalid = no blue line next to the letter C; the test must be repeated with a new cassette. If the problem continues, contact technical support.		
***Accurate Results** ______________ **Instructor Confirmation** ______________		

Follow-up: Postanalytical	**Scores**	
	S	**U**
*F. Proper documentation		
1. On control/patient log: ______________ yes ______________ no		
2. Documented on patient chart (see below).		
3. Identified critical values and took appropriate steps to notify physician		
- Expected values for analyte: negative for *H. pylori*		
G. Proper disposal and disinfection		
1. Disposed all sharps into biohazard sharps containers.		
2. Disposed all other regulated medical waste into biohazard bags.		
3. Disinfected test area and instruments according to OSHA guidelines.		
4. Sanitized hands after removing gloves.		
Total Points per Column		

Patient Name: ____

Patient Chart Entry: (Include when, what, how, why, any additional information, and the signature of the person charting.)

____

____

____

GENERIC ANALYTICAL TEST FORM (FOR KITS NOT COVERED IN THE TEXTBOOK OR WORKBOOK)

Qualitative Test: ______________________________

Person evaluated ______________________________ Date ______________________________

Evaluated by ______________________________ Score ______________________________

Outcome goal	
Conditions	Supplies required:
Standards	Required time = Performance time = ______________ Total possible points = ______________ Points earned = ______________
Evaluation Rubric Codes: **S** = Satisfactory, meets standard **U** = Unsatisfactory, fails to meet standard	
NOTE: Steps marked with an asterisk (*) are critical to achieve required competency.	

Preparation: Preanalytical Phase	**Scores**	
	S	**U**
A. Test information		
- Kit method:		
- Manufacturer:		
- Proper storage (e.g., temperature, light):		
- Lot # of kit: ______________________________		
- Expiration date: ______________________________		
- Package insert or test flow chart available ______________ yes ______________ no		
B. Personal protective equipment:		
C. Specimen information:		
Procedure: Analytical Phase	**Scores**	
	S	**U**
D. Performed/observed qualitative quality control		
- External liquid controls: positive ______________ negative ______________		
- Internal control		
E. Performed patient test		
1.		
2.		
3.		

4.		
Positive =		
Negative =		
Invalid =		
***Accurate Results** ________ **Instructor Confirmation** ________		
Follow-up: Postanalytical Phase	**Scores**	
	S	**U**
*F. Proper documentation		
1. On control/patient log: ________ yes ________ no		
2. Documented on patient chart (see below).		
3. Identified positive values and took appropriate steps to notify physician.		
G. Proper disposal and disinfection		
1. Disposed all sharps into biohazard sharps containers.		
2. Disposed all other regulated medical waste into biohazard bags.		
3. Disinfected test area and instruments according to OSHA guidelines.		
4. Sanitized hands after removing gloves.		
Total Points per Column		

Patient Name: ________________________________

Patient Chart Entry: (Include when, what, how, why, any additional information, and the signature of the person charting.)

____

____

____

8 Microbiology

VOCABULARY REVIEW

Match each definition with the correct term.

________ 1. malaise	A. Rate at which illness occurs
________ 2. myalgia	B. Having the pink or red color of the counterstain used in Gram's method of staining microorganisms
________ 3. expectoration	C. Diffuse muscle pain
________ 4. gram positive	D. Pertaining to unicellular organisms that do not have a true nucleus with a nuclear membrane
________ 5. fastidious	E. Retaining the purple color of the stain used in Gram's method of staining microorganisms
________ 6. mortality	F. Disease in the body caused by the invasion of pathogenic microorganisms
________ 7. gram negative	G. Coughing up sputum and mucus from the trachea and lungs
________ 8. infection	H. Component made of polysaccharides and peptides that gives rigidity to the bacterial cell wall
________ 9. peptidoglycan	I. Feeling of weakness, distress, or discomfort
________ 10. morbidity	J. Requiring special nutrients for growth
________ 11. eukaryotic	K. Pertaining to organisms that possess a true nucleus with a nuclear membrane and organelles
________ 12. prokaryote	L. Rate of deaths
________ 13. binary fission	M. Asexual reproduction in which the cell splits in half

FUNDAMENTAL CONCEPTS

14. Give an example of an organism that is normal flora, and discuss what can occur if the organism is destroyed.

____

____

15. Using Table 8-1 in the textbook, list two health issues of concern in the 1990s.

____

____

16. List two characteristics of bacteria.

____

____

17. Explain the difference between a yeast fungus and a mold fungus.

____

____

18. List the three general types of bacterial shapes, and give an example of each.

____

____

19. Match each bacterial shape or group with its name (see Figure 8-1 in the textbook).

_______ 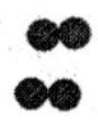 A. Bacilli

_______ 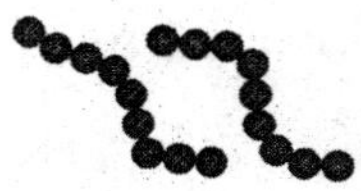 B. Spirilla

_______ 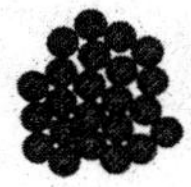 C. Streptococci

_______ 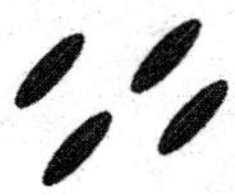 D. Staphylococci

_______ 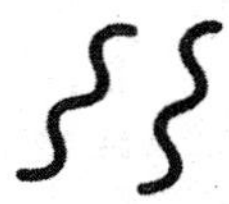 E. Diplococci

20. Describe the benefits that flagella, spores, and capsules give to organisms that possess these structures.

____

____

____

21. List four ways that a medical assistant can take precautions to prevent the spread of infection to others or to themselves.

____

____

22. When is the ideal time to collect a microbiology specimen?

____

____

23. Discuss the Jembec transport system.

____

____

24. Describe the cell wall structures that cause some organisms to be gram positive or gram negative.

____

____

25. Give the color of gram-positive and gram-negative organisms after the decolorizer step has been applied.

____

____

26. Label the supplies needed for Gram staining (see Procedure 8-2 in the textbook).

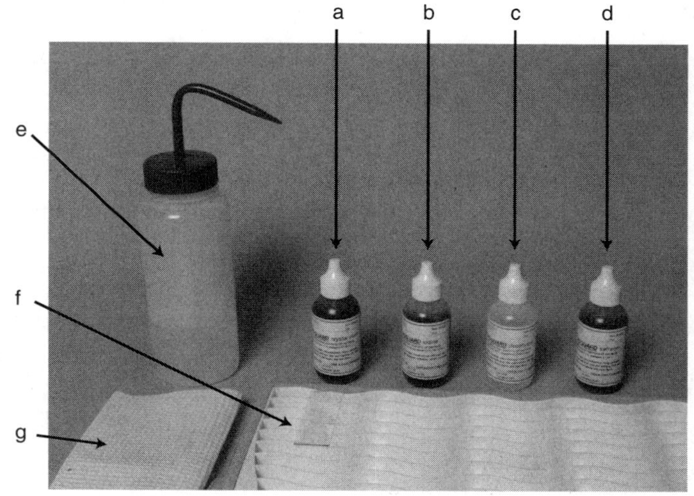

27. What is the causative agent for tuberculosis?

____

____

28. Describe the appearance and characteristics of *Trichomonas vaginalis*.

____

____

____

29. Case study: On each blank below, write **C** if the statement is correct and **I** if the statement is incorrect. If the step is incorrect, explain why in the space provided.
A medical assistant is performing Gram staining of a specimen.

_______ 1. The specimen is heat fixed to fix the specimen to the slide.

____

_______ 2. Crystal violet is applied to the slide for 2 minutes and then rinsed with water.

____

_______ 3. Gram's iodine is applied for 1 minute, and both gram-positive and gram-negative organisms are purple. Rinse with water.

____

_______ 4. The decolorizer is applied until the purple has stopped running off the slide. This is the most critical step. Rinse with water.

_______ 5. Safranin is applied last for 1 minute and rinsed with water. Gram-positive organisms are pink or red, and gram-negative organisms are purple.

PROCEDURES: CLINICAL LABORATORY IMPROVEMENT AMENDMENT (CLIA)–WAIVED MICROBIOLOGY TESTS

30. Describe the appearance of alpha, beta, and gamma hemolysis on blood agar plates.

31. State the causative agent (genus and species) of strep throat, and give the most common hemolytic reaction that this organism produces on blood agar plates.

32. What antibiotic is in the disk that is used to identify *Streptococcus pyogenes*?

33. Label the supplies needed to perform a group A *Streptococcus* test (see Procedure 8-5 in the textbook).

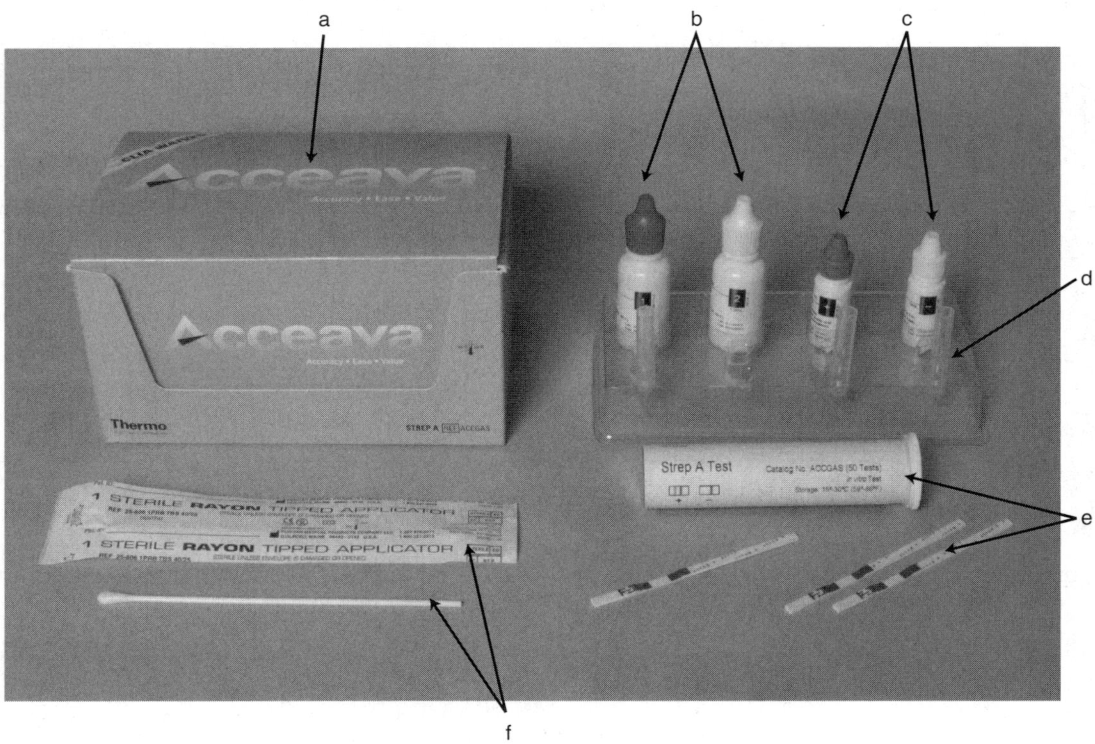

34. List three medical conditions associated with a strep infection.

35. When discussing influenza, what is the difference between antigenic *drift* and *shift*?

36. Describe how to obtain a nasal swab specimen when testing for influenza.

ADVANCED CONCEPTS

37. Give the oxygen requirements for aerobic, anaerobic, and facultative anaerobic organisms.

38. Name media requirements that most bacteria need for growth.

39. Explain how MacConkey media is a selective and a differential media.

40. Describe the shape, arrangement, and Gram stain appearance of *Neisseria gonorrhoeae*.

41. Give the advantages of using an incinerator instead of a Bunsen burner.

42. Describe or draw a picture of the differences between quadrant streaking and colony count streaking.

43. Explain a physician's reason for ordering a sensitivity test.

44. List three organisms that frequently cause urinary tract infections.

____

____

45. Case study: By using Tables 8-3 through 8-9 in the textbook, complete the following information:

Streptococcus pneumoniae

- Gram stain reaction: ____________________
- Disease: ____________________
- Transmission: ____________________
- Specimens: ____________________

Neisseria gonorrhoeae

- Gram stain reaction: ____________________
- Disease: ____________________
- Transmission: ____________________
- Specimens: ____________________

Chlamydia trachomatis

- Disease: ____________________
- Transmission: ____________________
- Specimens: ____________________

Enterobius vermicularis

- Transmission: ____________________
- Specimens or tests: ____________________

Urinary tract infections

- Organisms: ____________________
- Gram stain reaction: ____________________
- Transmission: ____________________
- Tests or specimen: ____________________

Food poisoning (most common cause in the United States)

- Organisms: ____________________
- Gram stain reaction: ____________________
- Transmission: ____________________
- Tests or specimen: ____________________

Procedure 8-1: Procedure for Collecting a Throat Specimen

Person evaluated ______________________ Date ______________

Evaluated by ______________________ Score ______________

Outcome goal	To perform throat specimen collection
Conditions	Supplies required: - Sterile swabs and tongue depressor - Personal protective equipment
Standards	Required time = 10 minutes Performance time = ________ Total possible points = ________ Points earned = ________
Evaluation Rubric Codes: **S** = Satisfactory, meets standard **U** = Unsatisfactory, fails to meet standard	
NOTE: Steps marked with an asterisk (*) are critical to achieve required competency.	

Preparation	**Scores** S	U
*1. Identified patient and placed in proper position.		
- Had patient state name.		
- Confirmed identification with patient.		
- Compared with requisition.		
Procedure	**Scores** S	U
*2. Sanitized hands and put on gloves and face mask.		
*3. Aseptically removed the sterile Dacron swab (cotton swab may inhibit growth of bacteria) from the package, holding only the tip of the swab.		
4. Had the patient sit with head back.		
*5. Used a sterile tongue depressor to hold down the tongue and had patient say "ahh."		
*6. Rotated the swab on the back of throat in a circular motion or figure-eight pattern.		
- Did not touch the teeth or back of the tongue because these areas have normal flora.		
- Two swabs can be used at the same time: one for a rapid strep test and one for a culture if needed.		
7. Inserted swab into appropriate container for testing.		
Follow-up	**Scores** S	U
8. Determined if patient was feeling well before dismissing.		
*9. Completed proper documentation on patient chart (see following page).		
*10. Proper disposal and disinfection		

- Disinfected test area and instruments according to OSHA guidelines.		
- Disposed regulated medical waste (e.g., gloves, tongue depressor) into biohazard bags.		
*11. Sanitized hands		
Total Points per Column		

Patient Name: ________________

Patient Chart Entry: (Include when, what, how, why, any additional information, and the signature of the person charting.)

____

____

Procedure 8-2: Gram Stain Procedure

Person evaluated ______________________ Date ______________

Evaluated by ______________________ Score ______________

Outcome goal	Perform a Gram stain
Conditions	Supplies required: - Gloves, bibulous paper, water bottle, or running water - Gram staining reagents: crystal violet, Gram's iodine, decolorizer, safranin - Staining rack
Standards	Required time = 15 minutes Performance time = ________ Total possible points = ________ Points earned = ________ Accuracy = final slide shows gram-positive and gram-negative bacteria
Evaluation Rubric Codes: **S** = Satisfactory, meets standard **U** = Unsatisfactory, fails to meet standard	

Preparation	Scores S	Scores U
1. Sanitized hands and applied gloves.		
2. Fixed specimen to the slide (using heat or methanol).		
Procedure	**S**	**U**
3. Applied crystal violet to slide for 1 minute.		
4. Rinsed slide with water.		
5. Applied Gram's iodine to slide for 1 minute.		
6. Rinsed slide with water.		
7. Poured decolorizer over the tilted slide until no more purple ran off (about 3–5 seconds) and then immediately rinsed slide with water to stop the reaction.		
8. Applied safranin stain for 1 minute.		
9. Rinsed slide with water.		
10. Blotted slide dry in absorbent bibulous paper.		
Follow-up	**S**	**U**
11. Proper disposal and disinfection		
- Disinfected test area and instruments according to OSHA guidelines.		
- Disposed regulated medical waste (e.g., gloves) into biohazard bags.		
- Sanitized hands.		
Total Points per Column		

Procedure 8-5: Acceava Strep A Test Procedure

Person evaluated ______________________________ Date ______________

Evaluated by ______________________________ Score ______________

Outcome goal	To perform FDA-approved, CLIA-waived rapid strep test following the most current OSHA safety guidelines and applying the correct quality control
Conditions	Supplies required: - Acceava rapid strep kit containing: - Reagent 1 and reagent 2 - Liquid controls, positive and negative - Soft plastic testing tubes - Test stick and its container - Sterile rayon swab taken from wrapper - Sterile tongue depressor - Gloves, face protection
Standards	Required time = 10 minutes Performance time = __________ Total possible points = __________ Points earned = __________
Evaluation Rubric Codes: **S** = Satisfactory, meets standard **U** = Unsatisfactory, fails to meet standard	
NOTE: Steps marked with an asterisk (*) are critical to achieve required competency.	

Preparation: Preanalytical Phase	**Scores**	
	S	**U**
A. Test information		
- Kit or instrument method: **Strep A Test**		
- Manufacturer: **Acceava**		
- Proper storage (e.g., temperature, light): **room temperature**		
- Lot # of kit: ______________________		
- Expiration date: ______________________		
- Package insert or test flow chart available: __________ yes __________ no		
B. Specimen information		
- Type of specimen: **throat swab using swab from kit (do not use cotton swabs)**		
C. Personal protective equipment: **gloves, facemask during throat swab, and biohazard container**		
Procedure: Analytical Phase	**Scores**	
	S	**U**
D. Performed/observed qualitative quality control		
- External liquid controls: positive __________ negative __________		
- Internal control: __________ (appears as a red line on test stick)		

E. Performed patient test	S	U
1. Sanitized hands and applied gloves.		
2. Just before testing, added three drops of reagent 1 and three drops of reagent 2 into the test tube. The solution should turn light yellow.		
3. Immediately put the throat swab into the extract solution.		
4. Vigorously mixed the solution by rotating the swab forcefully against the side of the tube at least 10 times. Best results are obtained when the specimen is vigorously extracted in the solution.		
5. Let stand for 1 minute, and then squeezed the swab with the sides of the tube as the swab was being withdrawn; discarded the swab into a biohazard container.		
6. Removed a test stick from the container and recapped immediately; placed the absorbent end of the test stick into the extracted sample in the tube.		
7. At 5 minutes, read and recorded the results.		
- Positive = a blue line in test area and pink line in control area, indicating the internal control worked.		
- Negative = no blue line in the test area and a pink line in control area, indicating the internal control worked.		
***Accurate Results** ____________ **Instructor Confirmation** ____________		

Follow-up: Postanalytical Phase	**Scores**	
	S	**U**
*F. Proper documentation		
1. On control/patient log: ____________ yes ____________ no		
2. Documented on patient chart (see below).		
3. Identified critical values and took appropriate steps to notify physician.		
- Expected values for analyte: negative for strep.		
G. Proper disposal and disinfection		
1. Disposed all sharps into biohazard sharps containers.		
2. Disposed all other regulated medical waste into biohazard bags.		
3. Disinfected test area and instruments according to OSHA guidelines.		
4. Sanitized hands after removing gloves.		
Total Points per Column		

Patient Name: ________________

Patient Chart Entry: (Include when, what, how, why, any additional information, and the signature of the person charting.)

____

____

____

Procedure 8-6: OSOM Influenza A and B Test Procedure

Person evaluated ______________________ Date ______________

Evaluated by ______________________ Score ______________

Outcome goal	To perform FDA-approved, CLIA-waived influenza test following the most current OSHA safety guidelines and applying the correct quality control
Conditions	Supplies required for the OSOM Influenza A&B Test: - Personal protective equipment (face mask and gloves) - Foam swab provided in kit to collect nasal specimen - Plastic testing tube provided in kit - Extract solution provided in kit - Testing strip provided in kit - Control swabs for influenza A and B - Container of testing strips with diagram showing how to interpret results
Standards	Required time = 10 minutes Performance time = ____________ Total possible points = ____________ Points earned = ____________
Evaluation Rubric Codes: **S** = Satisfactory, meets standard **U** = Unsatisfactory, fails to meet standard	
NOTE: Steps marked with an asterisk (*) are critical to achieve required competency.	

Preparation: Preanalytical Phase	Scores	
	S	**U**
A. Test information		
- Kit or instrument method: **OSOM A&B Influenza Test**		
- Manufacturer: **Genzyme**		
- Proper storage (e.g., temperature, light): **room temperature**		
- Lot # of kit: ______________________		
- Expiration date: ______________________		
- Package insert or test flow chart available: __________ yes __________ no		
B. Specimen information		
- Type of specimen: **nasal swab using swab from kit**		
- **Sanitize hands and apply gloves and facemask**		
- Insert the foam swab provided in the test kit into the patient's nostril displaying the most secretion. Using a gentle rotation, push the swab until resistance is met at the level of the turbinates (at least 1 inch into the nostril). Rotate the swab a few times against the nasal wall and gently rock it back and forth.		
C. Personal protective equipment: **gloves during testing**		

Procedure: Analytical Phase	Scores	
	S	U
D. Performed/observed qualitative quality control		
External swab controls: Positive A ____________ Positive B ____________		
- Negative A ____________ Negative B ____________		
- Internal control will appear as a blue line on test stick.		
E. Performed patient test	S	U
1. Sanitized hands and applied gloves.		
2. Placed the nasal swab into the plastic tube containing the designated amount of extraction buffer solution.		
3. Vigorously twisted the swab against the sides and bottom of the tube at least 10 times, which disrupted the virus particles and released the internal viral nucleoproteins into the solution.		
4. Extracted all the solution from the swab by squeezing the plastic tube against the swab while removing it from the tube and disposed of swab properly.		
5. Dipped the influenza test strip into the tube with the extraction buffer, making sure the arrows on the strip were pointing down.		
6. Allowed 10 minutes for migration of the solution across the test area and control area of the strip, which allowed the nucleoproteins from the virus to react with the reagents on the test strip, causing a color reaction.		
7. Read the results for the influenza A and B test.		
- Positive = Result showed a pink or purple line in the A or B test area and a pink line in the internal control area.		
- Negative = Result showed no color change in the A or B test area and a pink line in the internal control area.		
***Accurate Results** ____________ **Instructor Confirmation** ____________		

Follow-up: Postanalytical Phase	Scores	
	S	U
*F. Proper documentation		
1. On control/patient log: ____________ yes ____________ no		
2. Documented on patient chart (see following page).		
3. Identified critical values and took appropriate steps to notify physician.		
- Expected values for analyte: negative for influenza A and B		
G. Proper disposal and disinfection		
1. Disposed all sharps into biohazard sharps containers.		
2. Disposed all other regulated medical waste into biohazard bags.		
3. Disinfected test area and instruments according to OSHA guidelines.		
4. Sanitized hands after removing gloves.		
Total Points per Column		

Patient name: ________________

Patient Chart Entry: (Include when, what, how, why, any additional information, and the signature of the person charting.)

____

____

____

9 Toxicology

VOCABULARY REVIEW

Match each definition with the correct term.

_______ 1. idiosyncrasy	A. Methadone and morphine
_______ 2. pharmacokinetics	B. Blood carrying the drug through the body
_______ 3. opiates	C. Measurement that determines if a substance is present or absent
_______ 4. toxicity	D. Abnormal susceptibility to a drug or other agent that is peculiar to the individual
_______ 5. qualitative drug screening	E. Release of a prescribed drug from its dosage
_______ 6. absorption	F. Level at which a drug becomes poisonous in the body
_______ 7. liberation	G. Precise measurement of the amount of a substance present in the specimen
_______ 8. quantitative	H. Marijuana drug screening
_______ 9. buprenorphine	I. Passage of a substance through the surface of the body into body fluids and tissues
_______ 10. distribution	J. FDA-approved drug for treating opioid drug addiction
_______ 11. cannabinoid	K. Movement of drugs through the body from the time of introduction to elimination
_______ 12. metabolite	L. Substance produced by the metabolism of a drug in the body

FUNDAMENTAL CONCEPTS

13. List three reasons a specimen would be tested in a toxicology laboratory.

____

____

____

14. List three toxicology responsibilities in the ambulatory care setting.

____

____

____

15. Explain three ways an over-the-counter (OTC) drug can become toxic.

____

____

____

16. Define what makes a drug of abuse.

____

____

17. When testing for a drug, urine is usually used for a ____________ result, and blood is used for a ____________ result.

18. Describe *chain of custody* when processing a specimen for drug screening.

____

____

19. Define MRO.

____

____

20. Explain the results seen on the left side of the urine drug test illustration.

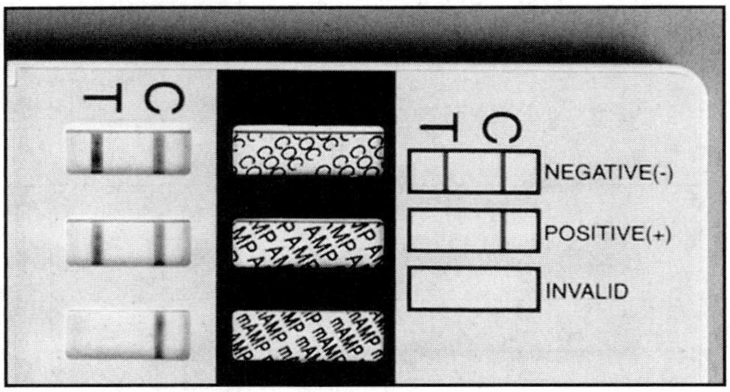

COC______________________________________

AMP______________________________________

mAMP ______________________________________

21. Using Table 9-1, write the drug name that matches the following testing codes:

THC______________________________________

COC______________________________________

BUP______________________________________

OPI ______________________________________

BAR______________________________________

BZO______________________________________

MTD______________________________________

AMP______________________________________

OXY______________________________________

mAMP ______________________________________

ADVANCED CONCEPTS

22. Why is it important to monitor drug levels during drug therapy?

____

____

23. From Table 9-4, list the six drug categories that require therapeutic monitoring.

____

____

24. Place the following pharmokinetic stages in order: metabolism, absorption, liberation, elimination, and distribution

____

____

25. Describe drug *half-life*.

____

26. List three environmental poisons that are tested in toxicology.

____

____

____

Procedure 9-1: Assisting with Urine Collection for Drug Screening

Person evaluated ______________________ Date ______________________

Evaluated by ______________________ Score ______________________

Outcome goal	To assist with urine collection for drug screening
Conditions	Supplies required: - Urine drug screening collection kit with specimen cup with temperature indicator - Urine specimen containers to be sent to the laboratory - Plastic sealable pouch for the two urine specimen containers chain of custody documents - Personal protective equipment
Standards	Required time = 15 minutes Performance time = __________ Total possible points = __________ Points earned = __________
Evaluation Rubric Codes: **S** = Satisfactory, meets standard **U** = Unsatisfactory, fails to meet standard	
NOTE: Steps marked with an asterisk (*) are critical to achieve required competency.	

Preparation	**Scores**	
	S	**U**
1. Explain to the patient the purpose of the test and the procedure to be followed for a midstream clean-catch specimen collection.		
- Had patient state name.		
- Obtained a signed consent form from the patient.		
- Compared with requisition.		
Procedure	**Scores**	
	S	**U**
2. Sanitized hands and put on gloves and face mask.		
3. A trained professional must witness the voiding of at least 50 mL of urine into the specimen cup provided in the urine collection drug kit.		
4. Originate the chain of custody document at the time of the sample collection. The person who witnessed the voiding must sign the document, as must every other person who handles the sample.		
5. After the collection, verify the temperature of the urine as seen on the indicator at the bottom of the cup, and document it. *Note:* If the temperature of the urine specimen is out of range (too cold), a second specimen must be collected. If the donor refuses to provide the second specimen under direct observation, the collection would be considered a "refusal to test."		
*6. Transfer the specimen to the two containers that must be labeled with the following information: • Full name of the patient • Date and time of collection • Your initials • Initials of the witnessing officer		

	S	U
7. Place the two sample containers into the sealed plastic pouch, mark it with a notary-style seal or with tamper-proof tape to protect the integrity of the sample, and send the specimen to the toxicology laboratory.		
8. Place the two sample containers into the sealed plastic pouch, mark it with a notary-style seal or with tamper-proof tape to protect the integrity of the sample, and send the specimen to the toxicology laboratory.		
9. If you are trained and qualified to do the testing, proceed with the testing according to laboratory and state regulations.		
Follow-up	**Scores**	
	S	**U**
10. After the initial and confirmatory testing is complete, mark the urine sample, reseal it, and securely store it for a minimum of 30 days or for the length of time specified by laboratory protocols.		
11. Completed proper documentation on patient chart (see below).		
12. Proper disposal and disinfection:		
- Disinfected test area and instruments according to OSHA guidelines. - Disposed regulated medical waste (e.g., gloves, tongue depressor) into biohazard bags.		
*13. Sanitized hands.		
Total Points per Column		

Patient Name: ________________________________

Patient Chart Entry: (Include when, what, how, why, any additional information, and the signature of the person charting.)

____

____

Procedure 9-2: Assisting with Blood Collection for Alcohol Testing

Person evaluated ______________________ Date ______________________

Evaluated by ______________________ Score ______________________

Outcome goal	To assist with blood collection for alcohol testing
Conditions	Supplies required: - Gray-topped Vacutainer tubes - Venipuncture needle and holder (or syringe and transfer device) - Nonvolatile disinfectant (e.g., benzalkonium [Zephiran], aqueous thimerosal [Merthiolate]) - Gauze - Tourniquet - Gloves - Legally authorized transportation envelope, container, or plastic pouch
Standards	Required time = 15 minutes Performance time = ______________ Total possible points = ______________ Points earned = ______________ Accuracy = final slide shows gram-positive and gram-negative bacteria
Evaluation Rubric Codes: **S** = Satisfactory, meets standard **U** = Unsatisfactory, fails to meet standard	
NOTE: Steps marked with an asterisk (*) are critical to achieve required competency.	

Patient Preparation	**Scores**	
	S	**U**
1. An officer of the law is present to act as a witness to the procedure.		
2. The patient probably is still under the influence of alcohol, so explain what you will be doing in as concise a manner as possible. *Note:* Do not allow yourself to become irritated by the speech or mannerisms of the patient. Treat the patient with the respect and dignity with which you treat all patients.		
Blood Collection Procedure	**Scores**	
	S	**U**
Note: The Department of Justice for each state has established uniform standards for the collection, handling, and preservation of blood samples used for alcohol testing. If you are authorized to obtain specimens for forensic analysis, check your laboratory's procedure manual so that you perform the collection *exactly* as required by the uniform standards established for your state.		
3. Sanitize hands, and apply gloves.		
4. Prepare the draw site using Zephiran, aqueous Merthiolate, or another aqueous disinfectant. *Do not use alcohol or other volatile organic disinfectants to clean the skin site.*		
5. Complete the blood draw, filling both tubes with sufficient blood to permit duplicate blood alcohol determinations.		

After Collection	Scores	
	S	U
6. Label the two gray-stoppered tubes with the following information: - Full name of the patient - Date and time of collection - Your initials - Initials of the witnessing officer		
7. Give the labeled blood samples to the witnessing officer, who will immediately complete the required information on the transportation envelope, container, or plastic pouch. The officer will then seal it securely. Information on the envelope or container should include the following: - The full name of the patient - Whether the patient is alive or dead - The submitting agency - The geographic location where the blood was drawn (e.g., hospital, clinic, jail) - The name of the person drawing the blood sample - The date and time the blood sample was drawn - The signature of the witnessing officer		
8. After the envelope or container is sealed, it must not be opened, except for analysis. Each person who is subsequently in possession of the sealed sample must sign his or her name in the space provided on the envelope or container (chain of custody). The integrity of the sample must be safeguarded.		
9. Remove gloves, and wash hands.		
Total Points per Column		

Procedure 9-3: Urine Drug Panel Testing Procedure

Person evaluated ______________________ Date ______________________

Evaluated by ______________________ Score ______________________

Outcome goal	To perform FDA-approved, CLIA-waived drug panel test following the most current OSHA safety guidelines and applying the correct quality control
Conditions	Supplies required: - Gloves - Test card with multiple test strips (five tests are on each side of the card) - Metal pouch containing the test card (check expiration date and temperature)
Standards	Required time = 10 minutes Performance time = ____________ Total possible points = ____________ Points earned = ____________
Evaluation Rubric Codes: **S** = Satisfactory, meets standard **U** = Unsatisfactory, fails to meet standard	
NOTE: Steps marked with an asterisk (*) are critical to achieve required competency.	

Preparation: Preanalytical Phase	**Scores**	
	S	**U**
A. Test information		
- Kit or instrument method:		
- Manufacturer:		
- Proper storage (e.g., temperature, light): stored the card at 2° to 30° C (check expiration date)		
- Lot # of kit: ____________		
- Expiration date: ____________		
- Package insert or test flow chart available: ____________ yes ____________ no		
B. Specimen information		
- Type of specimen: **Fresh urine specimen or specimen that has been stored at 2° to 8° C for up to 48 hours and then brought to room temperature.**		
C. Sanitize the hands, and apply gloves.		
Procedure: Analytical Phase	**S**	**U**
D. Performed/observed qualitative quality control		
- External liquid controls: positive ____________ negative ____________		
- Internal control: ____________ (appears as a red line on test stick)		

E. Performed patient test	S	U
1. Sanitize the hands, and apply gloves.		
2. Remove the test device from its protective pouch, and label it with the patient's identification. *Note*: If the specimen has been stored in the refrigerator, bring it to room temperature before opening to prevent condensation.		
3. Remove the cap from the end of the test card.		
4. With the arrows pointing toward the urine specimen, immerse the strips of the test card vertically into the urine specimen for at least 10 to 15 seconds. **Immerse the strips to at least the level of the wavy lines on the strips but not above the arrows on the test card.**		
5. Place the test card on a nonabsorbent surface, and wait for the colored lines to appear.		
6. At 5 minutes, read and record the results.		
- Positive test result: One distinct pink band appears in the control region (C), with no line in the test region (T).		
- Negative test result: Two pink bands appear, with one pink band in the control region (C) and one pink band in the patient test region (T).		
- Invalid: Pink bands are absent from the control region. Repeat the test with a new device. If the problem persists, call for technical assistance.		
***Accurate Results** ______________ **Instructor Confirmation** ______________		

Follow-up: Postanalytical Phase	**Scores**	
	S	**U**
*F. Proper documentation		
1. On control/patient log: ______________ yes ______________ no		
2. Documented on patient chart (see below).		
3. Identified critical values and took appropriate steps to notify physician.		
- Expected values for analyte: negative for strep		
G. Proper disposal and disinfection		
1. Disposed all sharps into biohazard sharps containers.		
2. Disposed all other regulated medical waste into biohazard bags.		
3. Disinfected test area and instruments according to OSHA guidelines.		
4. Sanitized hands after removing gloves.		
Total Points per Column		

Patient name: ____

Patient Chart Entry: (Include when, what, how, why, any additional information, and the signature of the person charting.)

____

____

____

Appendix: Forms for Documenting Safety, Quality Assurance, and CLIA Compliance

CONTENTS

LABORATORY TECH RESPONSIBILITIES

Full Name of Tech	Official Initials	Temp Check Date	Disinfected Counters	Other

MONTHLY LABORATORY MAINTENANCE LOG

Medical Clinic								
Daily Maintenance Control Chart								
Month	Year							
	Daily				Monthly			
Day	Refrig	Freezer	Room	Incubator	Bleach	Eye Wash	Shower	By
	2-8° C	0-20° C	15-30° C	34-36° C	Counters	Checked	Checked	
1								
2								
3								
4								
5								
6								
7								
8								
9								
10								
11								
12								
13								
14								
15								
16								
17								
18								
19								
20								
21								
22								
23								
24								
25								
26								
27								
28								
29								
30								
31								
Comments								

Exposure Event Number__________

Blood and Body Fluid Exposure Report Form

Facility name: ____________________

Name of exposed worker: Last: ____________ **First:** ____________ **ID#:** ________

Date of exposure: _____/_____/_____ **Time of exposure:** _____:_____ **AM** **PM** (Circle)

Job title/occupation: ____________ **Department/work unit:** ____________

Location where exposure occurred: ____________________

Name of person completing form: ____________________

Section I. Type of Exposure *(Check all that apply.)*

☐ **Percutaneous (Needle or sharp object that was in contact with blood or body fluids)**
(Complete Sections II, III, IV, and V.)

☐ **Mucocutaneous** *(Check below and complete Sections III, IV, and VI.)*
___ **Mucous Membrane** ___ **Skin**

☐ **Bite** *(Complete Sections III, IV, and VI.)*

Section II. Needle/Sharp Device Information

(If exposure was percutaneous, provide the following information about the device involved.)

Name of device: ____________________ ☐ Unknown/Unable to determine

Brand/manufacturer: ____________________ ☐ Unknown/Unable to determine

Did the device have a sharps injury prevention feature, i.e., a "safety device"?

☐ Yes ☐ No ☐ Unknown/Unable to determine

If yes, when did the injury occur?

☐ Before activation of safety feature was appropriate ☐ Safety feature failed after activation

☐ During activation of the safety feature ☐ Safety feature not activated

☐ Safety feature improperly activated ☐ Other: ____________

Describe what happened with the safety feature, e.g., why it failed or why it was not activated: ____________________

____

Section III. Employee Narrative *(Optional)*

Describe how the exposure occurred and how it might have been prevented:

____

____

____

NOTE: This is not a CDC or OSHA form. This form was developed by CDC to help healthcare facilities with detailed exposure information that is specifically useful for the facilities' prevention planning. Information on this page (#1) may meet OSHA sharps injury documentation requirements and can be copied and filed for purposes of maintaining a separate sharps injury log. Procedures for maintaining employee confidentiality must be followed.

(Courtesy of Centers for Disease Control and Prevention, http://www.cdc.gov/sharpssafety/pdf/AppendixA-7.doc)

Exposure Event Number__________

Section IV. Exposure and Source Information

A. **Exposure Details:** *(Check all that apply.)*

1. Type of fluid or material (For body fluid exposures only, check which fluid in adjacent box.)

☐ Blood/blood products
☐ Visibly bloody body fluid*
☐ Non-visibly bloody body fluid*
☐ Visibly bloody solution (e.g., water used to clean a blood spill)

***Identify which body fluid**

__ Cerebrospinal	__ Urine	__ Synovial
__ Amniotic	__ Sputum	__ Peritoneal
__ Pericardial	__ Saliva	__ Semen/Vaginal
__ Pleural	__ Feces/stool	__ Other/Unknown

2. Body site of exposure. *(Check all that apply.)*

☐ Hand/finger ☐ Eye ☐ Mouth/nose ☐ Face

☐ Arm ☐ Leg ☐ Other (Describe:____________________)

3. If percutaneous exposure:

Depth of injury *(Check only one.)*

☐ Superficial (e.g., scratch, no or little blood)
☐ Moderate (e.g., penetrated through skin, wound bled)
☐ Deep (e.g., intramuscular penetration)
☐ Unsure/Unknown

Was blood visible on device before exposure? ☐ Yes ☐ No ☐ Unsure/Unknown

4. If mucous membrane or skin exposure: *(Check only one.)*

Approximate volume of material

☐ Small (e.g., few drops)
☐ Large (e.g., major blood splash)

If skin exposure, was skin intact? ☐ Yes ☐ No ☐ Unsure/Unknown

B. **Source Information**

1. Was the source individual identified? ☐ Yes ☐ No ☐ Unsure/Unknown

2. Provide the serostatus of the source patient for the following pathogens.

	Positive	Negative	Refused	Unknown
HIV Antibody	☐	☐	☐	☐
HCV Antibody	☐	☐	☐	☐
HbsAg	☐	☐	☐	☐

3. If known, when was the serostatus of the source determined?

☐ Known at the time of exposure
☐ Determined through testing at the time of or soon after the exposure

Exposure Event Number__________

Section V. Percutaneous Injury Circumstances

A. **What device or item caused the injury?**

Hollow-bore needle

- ☐ Hypodermic needle
  - __ Attached to syringe __ Attached to IV tubing
  - __ Unattached
- ☐ Prefilled cartridge syringe needle
- ☐ Winged steel needle (i.e., butterfly type devices)
  - __ Attached to syringe, tube holder, or IV tubing
  - __ Unattached
- ☐ IV stylet
- ☐ Phlebotomy needle
- ☐ Spinal or epidural needle
- ☐ Bone marrow needle
- ☐ Biopsy needle
- ☐ Huber needle
- ☐ Other type of hollow-bore needle (type: ____)
- ☐ Hollow-bore needle, type unknown

Suture needle

- ☐ Suture needle

Glass

- ☐ Capillary tube
- ☐ Pipette (glass)
- ☐ Slide
- ☐ Specimen/test/vacuum
- ☐ Other: ______________________________

Other sharp objects

- ☐ Bone chip/chipped tooth
- ☐ Bone cutter
- ☐ Bovie electrocautery device
- ☐ Bur
- ☐ Explorer
- ☐ Extraction forceps
- ☐ Elevator
- ☐ Histology cutting blade
- ☐ Lancet
- ☐ Pin
- ☐ Razor
- ☐ Retractor
- ☐ Rod (orthopaedic applications)
- ☐ Root canal file
- ☐ Scaler/curette
- ☐ Scalpel blade
- ☐ Scissors
- ☐ Tenaculum
- ☐ Trocar
- ☐ Wire
- ☐ Other type of sharp object
- ☐ Sharp object, type unknown

Other device or item

- ☐ Other: ______________________________

B. **Purpose or procedure for which sharp item was used or intended.**
(Check one procedure type and complete information in corresponding box as applicable.)

- ☐ Establish intravenous or arterial access (Indicate type of line.) → Type of Line
- ☐ Access established intravenous or arterial line (Indicate type of line and reason for line access.) → Type of Line; Reason for Access
- ☐ Injection through skin or mucous membrane (Indicate type of injection.) → Type of Injection
- ☐ Obtain blood specimen (through skin) (Indicate method of specimen collection.) → Type of Blood Sampling
- ☐ Other specimen collection
- ☐ Suturing
- ☐ Cutting
- ☐ Other procedure
- ☐ Unknown

Type of Line

- __ Peripheral
- __ Central
- __ Arterial
- __ Other

Reason for Access

- __ Connect IV infusion/piggyback
- __ Flush with heparin/saline
- __ Obtain blood specimen
- __ Inject medication
- __ Other: ____________

Type of Injection

- __ IM Injection
- __ Skin test placement
- __ Other ID/SQ injection
- __ Epidural/spinal anesthesia
- __ Other injection

Type of Blood Sampling

- __ Venipuncture
- __ Arterial puncture
- __ Dialysis/AV fistula site
- __ Umbilical vessel
- __ Finger/heelstick
- __ Other blood sampling

Exposure Event Number__________

C. When and how did the injury occur? (From the left hand side of page, select the point during or after use that most closely represents when the injury occurred. In the corresponding right hand box, select *one* or *two* circumstances that reflect how the injury happened.)

☐ During use of the item →

Select one or two choices:

— Patient moved and jarred device
— While inserting needle/sharp
— While manipulating needle/sharp
— While withdrawing needle/sharp
— Passing or receiving equipment
— Suturing
— Tying sutures
— Manipulating suture needle in holder
— Incising
— Palpating/exploring
— Collided with co-worker or other during procedure
— Collided with sharp during procedure
— Sharp object dropped during procedure

☐ After use, before disposal of item →

Select one or two choices:

— Handling equipment on a tray or stand
— Transferring specimen into specimen container
— Processing specimens
— Passing or transferring equipment
— Recapping (missed or pierced cap)
— Cap fell off after recapping
— Disassembling device or equipment
— Decontamination/processing of used equipment
— During clean-up
— In transit to disposal
— Opening/breaking glass containers
— Collided with co-worker/other person
— Collided with sharp after procedure
— Sharp object dropped after procedure
— Struck by detached IV line needle

☐ During or after disposal of item →

Select one or two choices:

— Placing sharp in container:
  — Injured by sharp being disposed
  — Injured by sharp already in container
— While manipulating container
— Over-filled sharps container
— Punctured sharps container
— Sharp protruding from open container
— Sharp in unusual location:
  — In trash
  — In linen/laundry
  — Left on table/tray
  — Left in bed/mattress
  — On floor
  — In pocket/clothing
  — Other unusual location
— Collided with co-worker or other person
— Collided with sharp
— Sharp object dropped
— Struck by detached IV line needle

☐ Other (Describe): ______________________________

____

____

____

☐ Unknown

Exposure Event Number__________

Section VI. Mucous Membrane Exposures Circumstances

A. What barriers were used by worker at the time of the exposure? *(Check all that apply.)*

☐ Gloves ☐ Goggles ☐ Eyeglasses ☐ Face Shield ☐ Mask ☐ Gown

B. Activity/Event when exposure occurred *(Check one.)*

☐ Patient spit/coughed/vomited
☐ Airway manipulation (e.g., suctioning airway, inducing sputum)
☐ Endoscopic procedure
☐ Dental procedure
☐ Tube placement/removal/manipulation (e.g., chest, endotracheal, NG, rectal, urine catheter)
☐ Phlebotomy
☐ IV or arterial line insertion/removal/manipulation
☐ Irrigation procedure
☐ Vaginal delivery
☐ Surgical procedure (e.g., all surgical procedures including C-section)
☐ Bleeding vessel
☐ Changing dressing/wound care
☐ Manipulating blood tube/bottle/specimen container
☐ Cleaning/transporting contaminated equipment
☐ Other: ______________________________
☐ Unknown

Comments: ______________________________

GENERIC QUALITATIVE CONTROL AND PATIENT LOG (TEMPLATE)

Test: ______________________________

Kit Name and Manufacturer: ______________________________

Lot #: ______________________________ **Expiration Date:** ______________________________

Storage Requirements: ______________________________ **Test Flow Chart:** ______________________________

Date	Specimen ID (Control/Patient)	Result (+ or –)	Internal Control Passed (Y or N)	Charted in Patient Record	Tech Initials

GENERIC QUANTITATIVE TEST CONTROL LOG (TEMPLATE)

Control Lot #: ______________________ **Expiration Date** ______________________

Control Range: ______________________ **Control Level:** ______________________

Date	Tech	Result	Accept	Reject	Corrective Action

MONTHLY LEVY-JENNINGS QC CHART

Levy-Jennings Monthly Graph of Daily __________ Controls

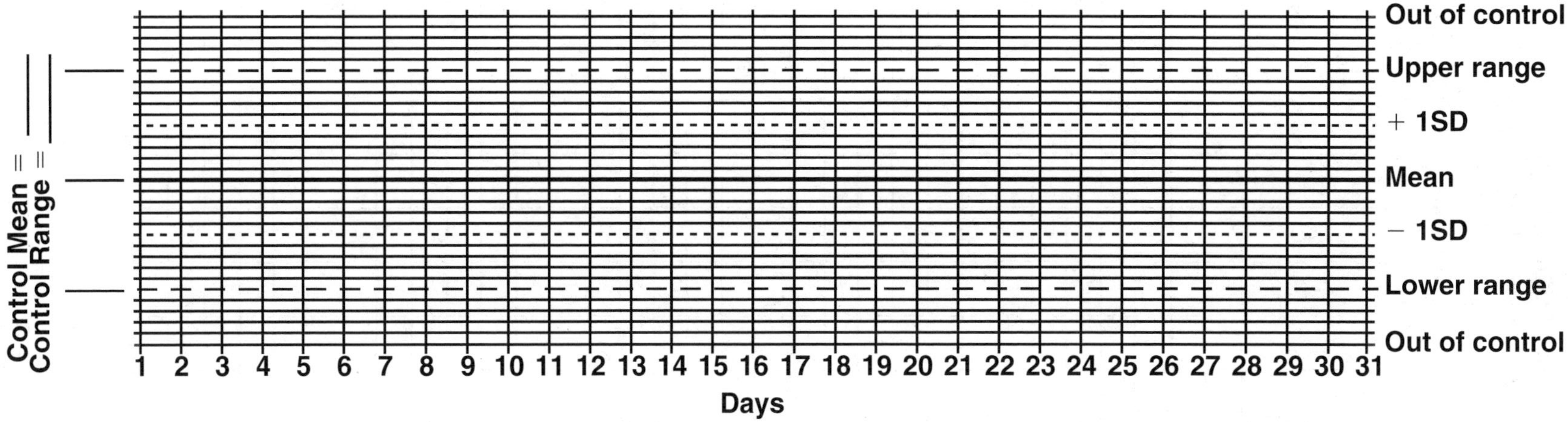

Levy-Jennings Monthly Graph of Daily __________ Controls

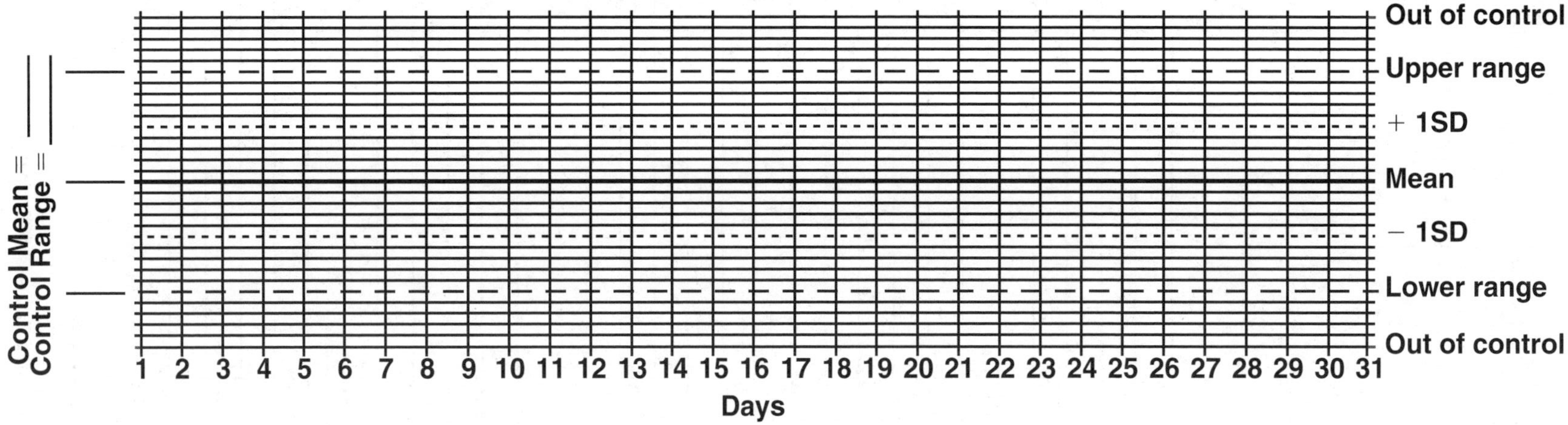

URINE DIPSTICK QUALITY CONTROL LOG

DATE__________ URINE DIPSTICK CONTROL LEVEL_________ LOT #__________ EXPIRATION DATE____________

		DIPSTICK TESTS										CONFIRMATORY TESTS				ADD. TESTS		
DATE	Reagent Strip Lot # Patient	Leukocytes	Nitrites	Urobilinogen	Protein	pH	Blood	Specific Gravity	Ketones	Bilirubin	Glucose	Protein Method/Lot #	Ketones Method/Lot #	Glucose Method/Lot #	Bilirubin Method/Lot #	hCG Method/Lot #	Specific Gravity Refractometer	INITIAL

(From Zakus SM: *Clinical skills for medical assistants*, ed 4, St. Louis, 2001, Mosby.)

URINE DIPSTICK PATIENT LOG

DATE	Reagent Strip / Lot# / Patient	DIPSTICK TESTS										CONFIRMATORY TESTS								ADD. TESTS			INITIAL
		Leukocytes	Nitrites	Urobilinogen	Protein	pH	Blood	Specific Gravity	Ketones	Bilirubin	Glucose	Protein	Method/Lot #	Ketones	Method/Lot #	Glucose	Method/Lot #	Bilirubin	Method/Lot #	hCG	Method/Lot #	Specific Gravity Refractometer	

(From Zakus SM: *Clinical skills for medical assistants*, ed 4, St. Louis, 2001, Mosby.)

Sample Device Pre-Selection Worksheet

Type of Device: ____________ Name: ____________ Manufacturer: ____________

	Clinical Considerations	Does this consideration apply to this device?		If Yes, what is the level of importance?		
		No	Yes	High	Med	Low
Procedural Implications for Healthcare Provider	Device use will require a change in technique (compared to conventional product).					
	Device permits needle changes.					
	Device permits reuse of the needle on the same patient during a procedure. (e.g., local anesthesia)					
	Device allows easy visualization of flashback.					
	Device allows easy visualization of medication.					
	Other:					
	Comment:					

Clinical Considerations		Does this consideration apply to this device?		If Yes, what is the level of importance?		
		No	Yes	High	Med	Low
Patient Considerations	Device is latex free.					
	Device has potential for causing infection.					
	Device has potential for causing increased pain or discomfort to patients.					
	Other:					
	Comment:					
Scope of Device Use Considerations	Device can be used with adult and pediatric populations.					
	Specialty areas (e.g., OR, anesthesiology, radiology) can use the device.					
	Device can be used for all same purposes for which the conventional device is used.					
	Device is available in all currently used sizes.					
	Other:					
	Comment:					

Safety Considerations		Does this consideration apply to this device?		If Yes, what is the level of importance?		
		No	Yes	High	Med	Low
Method Activation	The safety feature does not require activation by the user.					
	The worker's hands can remain behind the sharp during activation of the safety.					
	Activation of the safety feature can be performed with one hand.					
	Other:					
	Comment:					
Characteristics of the Safety Feature	The safety feature is in effect during use in the patient.					
	The safety feature permanently isolates the sharp.					
	The safety feature is integrated into the device (i.e., does not need to be added before use).					
	A visible or audible cue provides evidence of safety feature activation.					
	The safety feature is easy to recognize and intuitive to use.					
	Other:					
	Comment:					

Other Considerations		Does this consideration apply to this device?		If Yes, what is the level of importance?		
		No	Yes	High	Med	Low
Availability	The device is available in all sizes currently used in the organization.					
	The manufacturer can provide the device in needed quantities.					
Service Provided	The company representative will assist with training.					
	Product materials are available to assist with training.					
	The company will provide free samples for evaluation.					
	The company has a history of being responsive when problems arise.					
	Comment:					
Practical Considerations	The device will **not** increase the volume of sharps waste.					
	The device will **not** require changes in the size or shape of sharps containers.					
	Other:					
	Comment:					

Courtesy of Centers for Disease Control and Prevention, "Sample Device Pre-Selection Worksheet," Sharps Injury Prevention Workbook, A-12, http://www.cdc.gov/sharpssafety/index.html.

SAMPLE DEVICE EVALUATION FORM

Product: ______________________ **Date:** ______________________

Department/unit: ______________________ **Position/title:** ______________________

1. Number of times you used the device.

☐ **1–5** ☐ **6–10** ☐ **11–25** ☐ **26–50** ☐ **More than 50**

2. Please mark the box that best describes your experiences with the device. If a question is not applicable to this device, do not fill in an answer for that question.

Factors	Strongly Disagree	Disagree	Neither Agree nor Disagree	Agree	Strongly Agree
Patient/Procedure Considerations					
a. Needle penetration **is** comparable to the standard device.	1	2	3	4	5
b. Patients/residents **do not** perceive more pain or discomfort with this device.	1	2	3	4	5
c. Use of the device **does not** increase the number of repeat sticks of patient.	1	2	3	4	5
d. The device **does not** increase the time it takes to perform the procedure.	1	2	3	4	5
e. Use of the device **does not** require a change in procedural technique.	1	2	3	4	5
f. The device is compatible with other equipment that must be used with it.	1	2	3	4	5
g. The device can be used for the same purposes as the standard device.	1	2	3	4	5
h. Use of the device **is not** affected by my hand size.	1	2	3	4	5
i. Age or size of patient/resident **does not** affect use of this device.	1	2	3	4	5
Experience with the Safety Feature					
j. Safety feature **does not** interfere with procedural technique.	1	2	3	4	5
k. The safety feature is easy to activate.	1	2	3	4	5
l. Safety feature **does not** activate before the procedure is completed.	1	2	3	4	5
m. Once activated, the safety feature remains engaged.	1	2	3	4	5
n. I **did not** experience any injury or *near miss* of injury with the device.	1	2	3	4	5
Special Questions about this Particular Device					

[To be added by health care facility]	1	2	3	4	5
	1	2	3	4	5
	1	2	3	4	5
Overall Rating					
Overall, the device is effective for both patient/resident care and safety.	1	2	3	4	5

3. Did you participate in training on how to use this product?

☐ No *(Go to question 6.)* ☐ Yes *(Go to next question.)*

4. Who provided this instruction? *(Check all that apply.)*

☐ Product representative ☐ Staff development personnel ☐ Other ____________

5. Was the training you received adequate?

☐ No ☐ Yes

6. Was special training needed to use the product effectively?

☐ No ☐ Yes

7. Compared with others of your gender, how would you describe your hand size?

☐ Small ☐ Medium ☐ Large

8. What is your gender?

☐ Female ☐ Male

9. Which of the following do you consider yourself to be?

☐ Left-handed ☐ Right-handed

10. Please add any additional comments below.

____

____

THANK YOU FOR COMPLETING THIS SURVEY

Please return this form to:____

(Courtesy of Centers for Disease Control and Prevention, Sample Device Evaluation Form, Sharps Injury Prevention Workbook, A-13; http://www.cdc.gov/sharpssafety/index.html)

Quality Control Flow Chart for HemoCue

Regardless of the purpose, most clinical testing procedures have the same quality control requirements. If an instrument is used, there is usually a method to check its mechanical function. Often this is nothing more than an "optic check" or calibration strip supplied with the instrument to allow the user to determine whether the instrument is functional.

After determining that the instrument does indeed function, one then needs to prove that the reagents will perform as expected. Commonly, one uses a high and low value control sample. Look at the results. Are they within their expected ranges? If so, you can begin to test patients. If not, then it is time to do some troubleshooting.

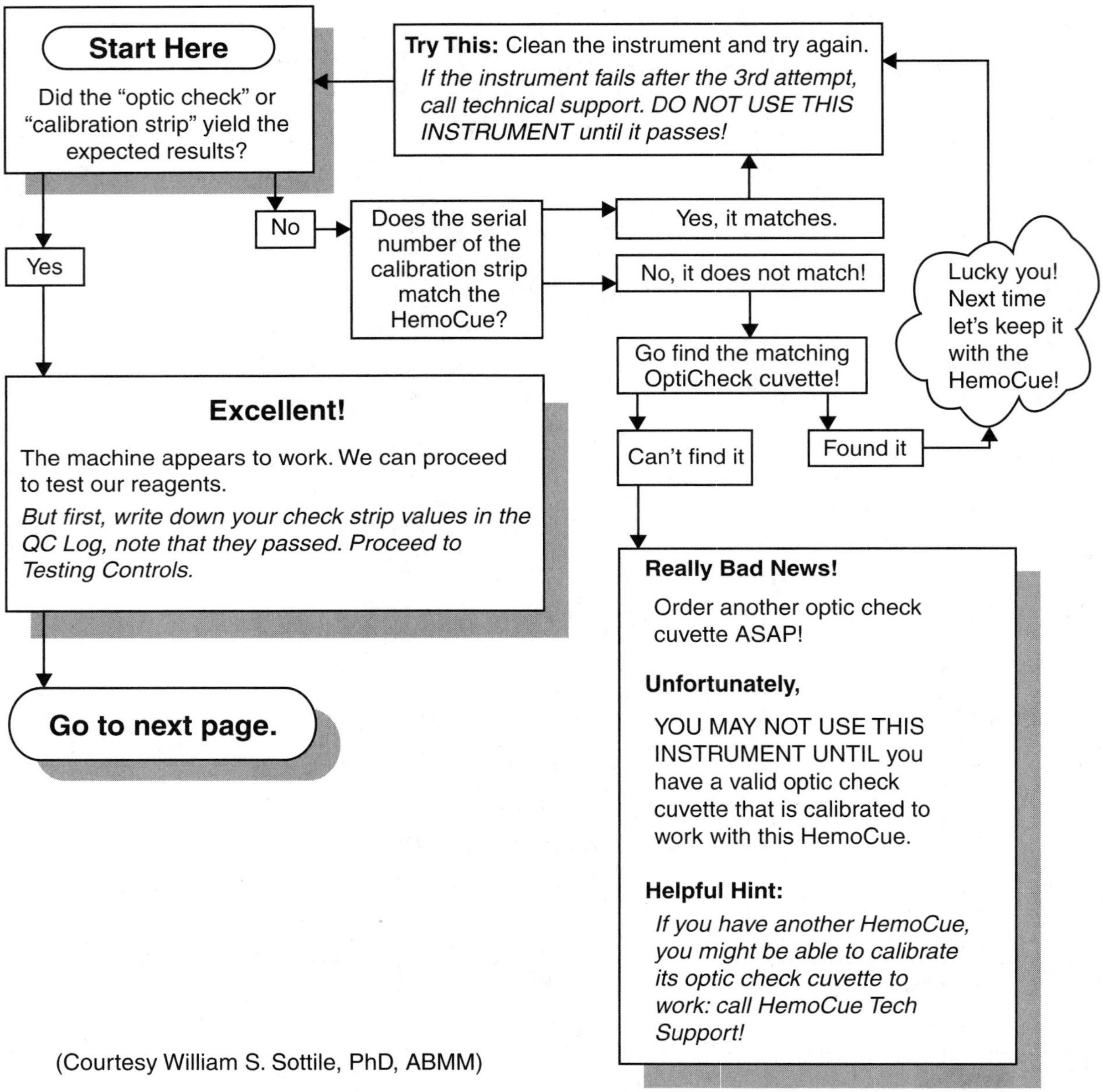

(Courtesy William S. Sottile, PhD, ABMM)

HEMOGLOBIN QUALITY CONTROL LOG

Test: ______________________________ **Control Lot #:** ______________________________

Control Range: ______________________________ **For Low/Normal/High Control**

Date	Tech	Result	Accept	Reject	Corrective Action

HEMOGLOBIN PATIENT LOG

Test: ______________________ **Kit Lot #:** ______________________

Expected Hemoglobin Values:

Adult males = 13.0–18 g/dL **Adult females = 11.0–16.0 g/dL**

Infants = 10.0–14.0 g/dL **Children = Increase to adult**

Date	Tech	Patient ID	Result	Charted

HEMATOCRIT QUALITY CONTROL LOG

Test: ______________________________ **Control Lot #:** ____________________

Control Range : ______________________ **For Low/Normal/High Control**

Date	Tech	Slot #	Result	Accept	Reject	Corrective Action

HEMATOCRIT PATIENT LOG

Expected Hematocrit Values:

Adult males = 42–52% | **Adult females = 36–48%**

Infants = 32–38% | **Children = Increase to adult**

Date	Tech	Patient ID	Slot #	Result	Charted

ERYTHROCYTE SEDIMENTATION RATE PATIENT LOG

Expected ESR Values:

Adult males < 50 yr = 0–15 mm/hr **Adult females < 50 yr = 0–20 mm/hr**

Adult males > 50 yr = 0–20 mm/hr **Adult females > 50 yr = 0–30 mm/hr**

Date	Tech	Patient ID	Slot #	Time	Result	Charted

PROTIME PATIENT LOG

ProTime expected values for normal and therapeutic whole blood:

	INR	PT (seconds; see ranges in insert)
Normal	0.8–1.2	________________
Low anticoagulation	1.5–2.0	________________
Moderate anticoagulation	2.0–3.0	________________
High anticoagulation	2.5–4.0	________________

Date	Tech	Patient ID	INR	PT (seconds)	Charted

GLUCOSE TEST CONTROL LOG

Control Lot #: ______________________ **Expiration Date:** ______________________

Control Range: ______________________ **Level: Low/Normal/High**

Date	Tech	Result	Accept	Reject	Corrective Action

GLUCOSE PATIENT LOG

Date	Patient	Result	Charted	Tech

HEMOGLOBIN A1c PATIENT/CONTROL LOG

Date	Patient	Result	Charted	Tech

CHOLESTECH LDX PATIENT/CONTROL LOG

____

Cassette Lot #: ____________ **Expiration Date:** ____________ **LDX Serial #:** ____________

Date	Operator	Patient ID	Charted	TRG	TC	GLU	HDL	LDL	TC/ HDL	ALT

HEMOCCULT PATIENT LOG

Date	Patient	Result	Tech

I-STAT PATIENT/CONTROL LOG

Cartridge Lot #: ____________ **Expiration Date:** ____________ **Serial #:** ____________

Date	Operator	Patient ID	Charted	Na	K	Cl	TCO_2	iCa	Glu	BUN	Crea	Hct	Hb	AnGap

Levy-Jennings Monthly Graph of Daily __________ Controls

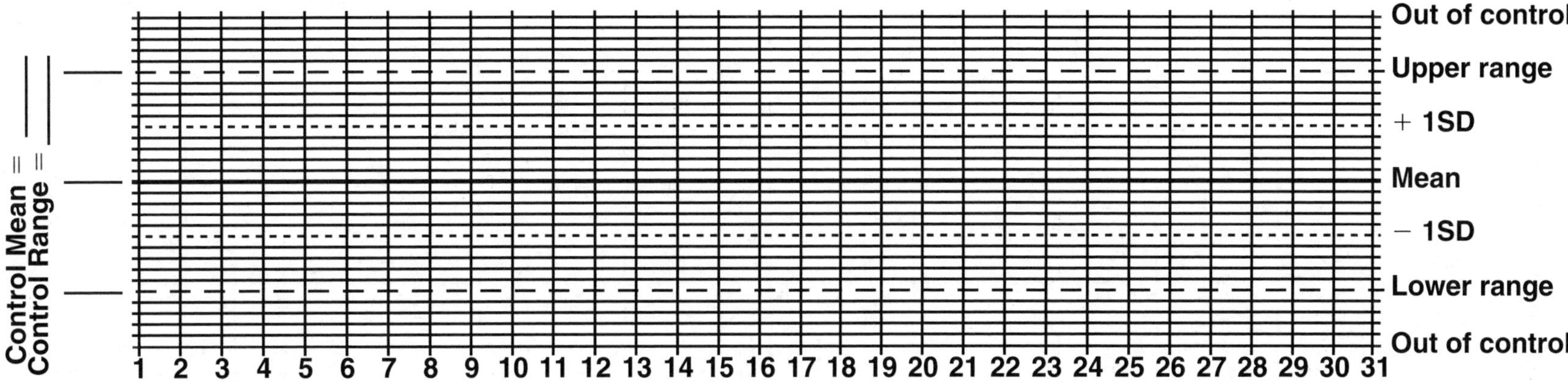

Levy-Jennings Monthly Graph of Daily __________ Controls

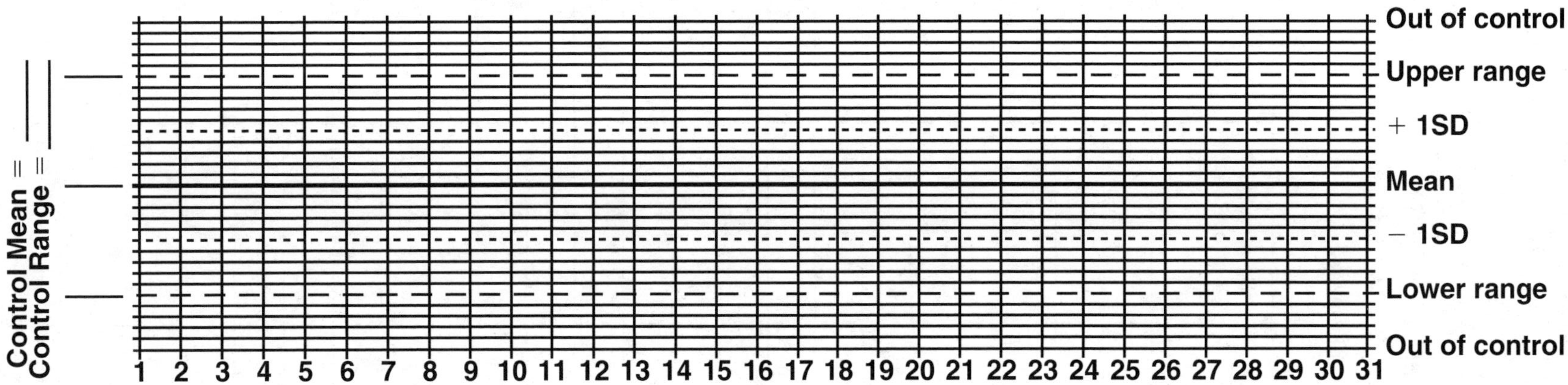

QUALITATIVE CONTROL AND PATIENT LOG FOR IMMUNOLOGY AND MICROBIOLOGY TEST KITS (TEMPLATE)

Test: ____________________

Kit Name and Manufacturer: ____

Lot # ____________________ **Expiration Date:** ____________________

Storage Requirements: ____________________ **Test Flow Chart:** ____________________

Date	Specimen ID (Control/Patient)	Result (+ or –)	Internal Control Passed (Y or N)	Charted in Patient Record	Tech Initials

GENERIC QUALITATIVE TEST PROCEDURE (TEMPLATE)

Qualitative Test ______________________________

Person evaluated ______________________________ **Date** ____________________

Evaluated by ______________________________ **Score** ____________________

Outcome goal:	Supplies required:
Conditions:	Required time = __________ minutes Performance time = __________
Standards:	Total possible points = __________ Points earned = __________
Evaluation Rubric Codes: **S** = Satisfactory - Meets standard **U** = Unsatisfactory - Fails to meet standard	
NOTE: Steps marked with an asterisk (*) are critical to achieve required competency.	

Preparation: Preanalytical Phase	**Scores**	
	S	**U**
A. Test information		
- Kit method:		
- Manufacturer:		
- Proper storage (e.g., temperature, light):		
- Lot number of kit: __________________		
- Expiration date: __________________		
- Package insert and/or test flow chart available: __________ yes __________ no		
B. Personal protective equipment		
C. Specimen information		

Procedure: Analytical Phase	**Scores**	
	S	**U**
D. Performed/observed qualitative quality control		
- External liquid controls: Positive __________ Negative __________		
- Internal control:		
E. Performed patient test	**S**	**U**
1.		
2.		
3.		
4.		

	S	U
POSITIVE seen as:		
NEGATIVE seen as:		
INVALID seen as:		
***Accurate Results** ____________ **Instructor Confirmation** ____________		
Follow-up: Postanalytical Phase	**Scores**	
	S	**U**
*F. Proper documentation		
1. On control/patient log: ____________ yes ____________ no		
2. Documentation on patient chart (see below).		
3. Identified "critical values" and took appropriate steps to notify physician EXPECTED VALUES FOR ANALYTE: NEGATIVE		
G. Proper disposal and disinfection		
1. Disposed all sharps into biohazard sharps containers.		
2. Disposed all other regulated medical waste into biohazard bags.		
3. Disinfected test area and instruments according to OSHA guidelines.		
4. Sanitized hands after removing gloves.		
Total Points per Column		

Patient Name: ____________________

Patient Chart Entry: (Include when, what, how, why, any additional information, and the signature of the person charting.)

____

____

____

GENERIC QUANTITATIVE TEST PROCEDURE (TEMPLATE)

Qualitative Test ______________________

Person evaluated ______________________ **Date** ______________

Evaluated by ______________________ **Score** ______________

Outcome goal:	
Conditions:	
Standards:	Required time = ________ minutes Performance time = ________ Total possible points = ________ Points earned = ________

Evaluation Rubric Codes:
S = Satisfactory - Meets standard **U** = Unsatisfactory - Fails to meet standard

NOTE: Steps marked with an asterisk (*) are critical to achieve required competency.

Preparation: Preanalytical Phase	**Scores**	
	S	**U**
A. Test information		
- Kit or instrumental method: ________		
- Manufacturer: ________		
- Proper storage (e.g., temperature, light): ________		
- Lot number of kit or supplies: ________		
- Expiration date: ________		
- Package insert and/or test flow chart available: ________ yes no ________		
B. Specimen information		
- Type of specimen and its preparation (e.g., fasting, first morning): ________		
- Specimen container or testing device: ________		
- Amount of specimen: ________		
C. Personal protective equipment (PPE): ________		
D. Assembled all the above, sanitized hands, and applied PPE		
Procedure: Analytical Phase	**Scores**	
	S	**U**
E. Performed/observed quality control		
Quantitative testing controls		
- Calibration check: ________		
- Control levels: Normal ________ High ________ Low ________		

F. Performed patient test: Followed proper steps (see flow chart and list steps)	S	U
1.		
2.		
3.		
4.		
5.		
6.		
7.		
8.		
9.		
10.		
***Accurate Results** ____________ **Instructor Confirmation** ____________		
Follow-up: Postanalytical	**Scores**	
	S	**U**
*G. Proper documentation		
1. On control log ____________ yes ____________ no		
2. On patient log ____________ yes ____________ no		
3. Documentation on patient chart (see below)		
4. Identified "critical values" and took appropriate steps to notify physician EXPECTED VALUES FOR ANALYTE:		
H. Proper disposal and disinfection		
1. Disposed all sharps into biohazard sharps containers		
2. Disposed all other regulated medical waste into biohazard bags		
3. Disinfected test area and instruments according to OSHA guidelines		
4. Sanitized hands after removing gloves		
Column Totals		

Patient Chart Entry: (Include when, what, how, why, any additional information, and the signature of the person charting.)

____

____

____

PROFESSIONAL EVALUATION FORM FOR THE LABORATORY CLASSROOM

Student: ____________________ **Date:** ____________________

Class: ____________________ **Semester:** ____________________

Number of Tardies: ____________________ **Number of Hours Absent:** ____________________

Objective	Very Satisfactory 3	Satisfactory 2	Unsatisfactory 1	Comments
Exhibits professional written communication (e.g., appearance, language, grammar).				
Uses the class materials appropriately (e.g., equipment, supplies, computers, cleanup).				
Provides instructor with all necessary information in a timely and organized manner (e.g., meets due dates, make-ups turned in within a week).				
Adheres to specific course policies (e.g., make-up guidelines, skill check-offs, externship guidelines).				
Projects a positive attitude and motivation (e.g., seen during lectures and labs).				
Displays professional verbal communication at all times (e.g., respectful, tactful).				
Maintains confidentiality of all personal interactions at all times (see rules of confidentiality in handbook).				
Projects professional work ethics (e.g., responsible, accountable, independent, full use of lab time: practice, study, computer).				
Cooperates with fellow students (e.g., team projects, skill practice, study groups).				
Displays responsible attendance behavior (e.g., arriving on time, calling in if detained or absent, prepared for next class session).				
Dresses appropriately (see handbook).				

Additional Comments:

____

____

____

Student Signature ____________________ **Instructor** ____________________

SAMPLE HEALTH ASSESSMENT FORM

Please print clearly: Date ______________

Name ______________ Address ______________

City ______________ State ______ ZIP ______

Telephone ______________ Age (date of birth) ____/ ____/ ____

Sex ______ Race ______ Ht. ______ Wt.______

Do you consider yourself overweight? ______ If so, how much? ______

Name of family doctor ______________ When last seen? ______________

Do you smoke? ______ If yes, how many packs per day ______ Alcohol use? ______

Do you have ____ Heart trouble ____ High blood pressure

____ Kidney problems ____ Heart attack before/ after 40

Are you taking medication for cholesterol? ____ Blood pressure? ______ Other? ______

Do you exercise regularly?______ When did you last eat? ______ hours

When you are finished with all your tests, please return to this room for final review of your results.

RELEASE:

I RELEASE ______________ and the Health Technology Students from any liability as a result of my participation in this free Health Fair.

Signature ______________ Date ______

Parent/Guardian ______________ Witness ______________

TEST	NORMAL LIMITS	RESULTS	FURTHER EVALUATION ______

URINALYSIS ☐

Glucose	NEG	
Bilirubin	NEG	
Ketone	NEG	
Specific gravity	1.005–1.030	
Blood	NEG	
pH	6.0–8.0	
Protein	NEG/TRACE	
Urobilinogen	NORM	
Nitrite	NEG	
Leukocytes	NEG	

Clinitek: asterisk (*) indicates further evaluation

Urinalysis

Routine urinalysis is a basic test, but it provides the physician with a tremendous amount of information about a disease. This test can help confirm or rule out a suspected diagnosis. It is a routine test that is repeated annually or as frequently as necessary to evaluate the patient's health status.

HEMATOLOGY

Anemia Hemoglobin: greater than 12 gm or g/dL ______ ☐

Hematocrit: greater than 32% ______ ☐

Anemia Check

The hemoglobin and hematocrit tests determine the oxygen-carrying ability of the blood. They are simple and efficient methods to detect any anemia. A patient is considered anemic if the hemoglobin value is below 12 mg/dL or the hematocrit is below 34%. Low values are caused by hemorrhage, pregnancy, recent menstruation, iron deficiency, or other causes that the physician needs to evaluate.

Erythrocyte Sedimentation Rate (ESR) = 0–20 mm/hr ______ ☐

Erythrocyte sedimentation rates are increased in infectious and inflammatory diseases, tissue destruction, and other conditions that increase the plasma fibrinogen level.

COAGULATION

INRatio ____________ INR ☐

ProTime ____________ seconds

> Desirable 0.8–1.2 INR
>
> Therapeutic 1.5–4.0 INR
>
> PT = seconds

BLOOD CHEMISTRY

Glucose **Fasting** ____________ (8 or more hours since eating) ☐

Random (hours since eating) ____________ hr

Normal 80–125 mg/dL (if 2 hr after eating) ____________

Hemoglobin A_{1c} **Desirable levels are below 7%** **Result** ____________

WARNING SIGNS OF DIABETES	
Type 1 Diabetes	**Type 2 Diabetes**
Constant urination Abnormal thirst Unusual hunger Rapid loss of weight Irritability Obvious weakness or fatigue Nausea and vomiting	Drowsiness Itching A family history of diabetes Blurred vision Excessive weight Tingling, numbness in feet Easy fatigue Skin infections and slow healing

LIPID PROFILE (CHOLESTECH TEST)

Lipid Profile	Desirable Numbers	Cholestech Results
Total cholesterol	Less than 200 mg/dL	
HDL cholesterol	Greater than 40 mg/dL	
LDL cholesterol	Less than 130 mg/dL	
Triglycerides	Less that 150 mg/dL	
TC/HDL ratio	4.5 or less	
Glucose	Fasting: 60-110 mg/dL	
	Nonfasting: less than 160 mg/dL	

Cholesterol

Cholesterol measurements are used to diagnose and monitor disorders involving excess cholesterol in the blood and fat metabolism disorders. These conditions often are associated with coronary heart disease. It is thought that lowering mean cholesterol levels can reduce coronary heart disease.

CHEMISTRY PROFILE I-STAT (Chem 8+)

Test	Test Symbol	Units	Reference Range	Result
Sodium	Na	mmol/L	138–146	
Potassium	K	mmol/L	3.5–4.9	
Chloride	Cl	mmol/L	98–109	
Total carbon dioxide	TCO_2	mmol/L	24–29	
Ionized calcium	iCa	mmol/L	1.12–1.32	
Glucose	Glu	mg/dL	70–105	
Urea nitrogen	BUN	mg/dL	8–26	
Creatinine	Crea	mg/dL	0.6–1.3	
Hematocrit	Hct	% PCV	38–51	
Hemoglobin*	Hb	g/dL	12–17	
Anion gap*	AnGap	mmol/L	10–20	

FECAL OCCULT BLOOD

Results: Positive ____________ **Negative** __________________